Make the Connection

Make the Connection

TEN STEPS TO A BETTER BODY
–and a better life

BOB GREENE AND
OPRAH WINFREY

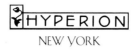

NEW YORK

Copyright © 1996, Harpo, Inc., and Bob Greene and Oprah Winfrey

Illustrations by Julie Johnson

Library of Congress Cataloging-in-Publication Data

Greene, Bob (Bob W.)
Make the connection : ten steps to a better body and a better life
/ by Bob Greene and Oprah Winfrey. — 1st ed.
p. cm.
ISBN 0-7868-6256-4
1. Physical fitness. 2. Physical fitness—Physiological aspects.
3. Health.—I. Winfrey, Oprah. II. Title.
GV481.G746 1996
613.7—dc20   96-8067
CIP

Paperback ISBN: 0-7868-8298-0

Designed by Claudyne Bianco Bedell

FIRST PAPERBACK EDITION

10 9 8 7 6 5 4 3 2 1

Contents

Foreword

SINCE the original publication of *Make the Connection* in September of 1996, a number of new, "revolutionary" methods to help you lose weight have been introduced. There seems to be no limit to the ways in which you can shed pounds. There are your basic theme diets, exercise programs, equipment gadgets, dietary supplements, and breakthrough drugs. Yes, your choices are virtually endless—you can eat cabbage, bust sugar, live in the "zone." You can go on the revolutionary Atkins diet (again), on the seven-day fat-burning program, or you can "spare protein in a modified fasting" kind of way. You can go on a liquid diet, or a liquid diet only on weekends; eat-fruit-only for breakfast, eat fruit only for lunch, or subscribe to the very original eat-fruit-only for dinner regimen.

You can go on one of the diets that tell you to eat only one primary "staple" food—just pick one from the following list: celery, jellybeans, lettuce, Tabasco sauce, gum or chocolate. There are the carbohydrates-only-at-breakfast, carbohydrates-only-at-lunch, and the carbohydrates-only-for-dinner plans. And, of course, the zero-carbohydrate program, even though your brain needs a certain amount of carbohydrates to function properly—oh well, mental acuity is really overrated anyway. Some of these plans have other minor side effects, but hey, gas and bad breath are a small price to pay for being more attractive.

If you're over the diet thing, you could try a hot new exercise program. You can go on one of the celebrity regimens—just pick your favorite celeb—or you can always sweat to the oldies. If there's a "problem area" you're concerned with, you can select one of the many exercise gadgets available. There's the various "ab" exercisers, infamous thigh machine, or the "you name your problem spot and we'll turn it to steel" tapes—to name just a few.

Of course, with exercise, you may just have to break a sweat. Perhaps you should simply take a supplement or two. Just one in the morning, and your life is suddenly much better. There's chromium, DHEA, and a multitude of other supplements. Okay, you tried that routine and your life wasn't all that much better—how about something a little stronger? How about a prescription? Of course, Fenfluramine got axed from the marketplace since it was found to cause damage to your heart. Or you could always just wait—there's bound to be another miracle sometime soon.

Right about now, I know you're waiting for the clincher, the punch line, the sentence that tells you that it's all nonsense. Actually, virtually all of the previously stated ways to drop unwanted pounds will make most people lose weight. In the short term, at the very least. And we all want to believe that there is some secret or magic with whatever plan we're following.

Here's the secret: When we are on any plan, we tend to be more conscious about what we eat and the amount of exercise we perform, and we lose weight. But when the specifics of the plan become too difficult or unreasonable to follow for a lifetime, we go off the plan, stop losing weight, lose motivation and start looking for the next miracle. We all know someone who has tried one of these gimmicks or plans, and has been successful. It's virtually always because—once they stopped using the "miracle" plan—they adopted a sensible program of moderate eating and regular exercise.

The flood of new ways to lose weight will continue. Do you know that we spend an estimated 35 to 40 billion dollars a year trying to lose weight? And there's no end in sight. One thing you can count on—if someone will buy it, it will be sold.

This feeding frenzy about weight loss products will continue as long as people are desperate to lose weight and are looking for a miracle answer. And don't let me off the hook, either—after all, this is a book partially about weight loss. I do, however, think that you'll find that there's a lot of good, truthful information here.

Oprah and I wanted to show you a healthy way to live your life. We wanted to tell you that it's not about shedding pounds; it's about feeling better about yourself. At some point, I hope you will understand that this is not simply a book about weight loss; this is a book about living a healthy life, eliminating behaviors that are contrary to your best interest, and developing a positive image of yourself. We hope at the very least you will understand that there is no value in being desperate to lose weight and there's no miracle answer aside from the power within you, the human desire and drive to better yourself.

For many people, losing weight is a journey of self-discovery. This book tells just such a story. It just happens to be the journey of a very public person, whose life is dedicated to inspiring others.

—Bob Greene

*A*nd the nominees for Best Talk-Show Host are . . ." Those five seconds when the announcer is calling your name—no matter who you are or what you've been told about what an honor it is to be nominated—at that moment, when your name is announced before the world, you want to win. Except for me, this night. I honestly didn't care.

I was sitting in the front row trying to keep my too-fat knees together in a ladylike position. But I'd never sat in this skirt before. And although it was just above knee-length standing, when I sat down, it did too. It was much too short for a fat woman, sitting in the front row with a camera eyeing my every move.

"I shouldn't have come," I thought. "I just shouldn't have come. I should have sent a message that I was sick. I should have worn a longer dress. I should have lost weight."

As they were running the video presentation of each host's show, I was thinking of whom I would like to see win instead of me. "Phil," I hoped. "Yes, God, let Phil win. So I won't have to get up and pull my skirt down and waddle my way up to the stage with the nation watching my huge behind."

I was 237 pounds—the fattest I'd ever been. The weight was consuming me. Even at what was supposed to be one of the most fulfilling and rewarding moments in my life, being honored at the Daytime Emmy Awards by my peers and the public for a job well done, all I could think about was how fat I was and how glamorous all the soap stars looked.

I hated my outfit. I was wearing a too-short, gold silk skirt and combination bronze-and-gold dinner jacket that had been tailor-made for me. Andre, who does my hair and wardrobe, had tried to convince me to wear something else. "Something more slimming," he said. "I don't care," I told

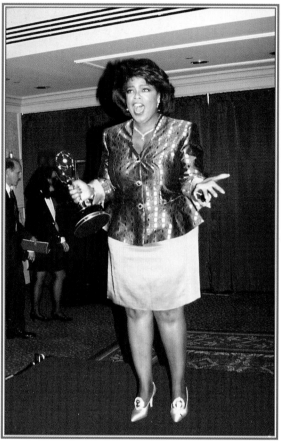

JUDIE BURSTEIN

him. *"How can you look slimmer when you're 237 pounds? Who am I trying to fool?"* Now I wished I'd listened to him. I should have worn black. I wished I could disappear.

"And the winner is Oprah Winfrey." I was stunned. Stedman and my staff were cheering. I wanted to cry. Not because I won, but because I would now have to stand before this audience of beautiful people and be judged. And not for being a winner.

I felt so much like a loser, like I'd lost control of my life. And the weight was symbolic of how out-of-control I was. I was the fattest woman in the room.

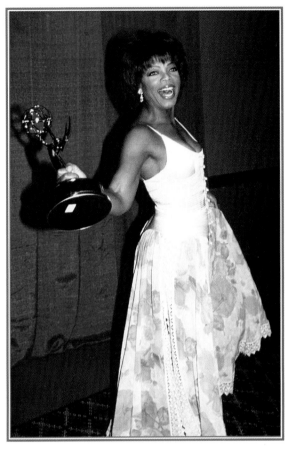

RETNA LTD.

The next day I met Bob. That's when my life began to change.

Up until that point I had spent a lifetime dieting and depriving myself, then overeating and gaining even more weight. It all started when I arrived in Baltimore at the age of 22. I had a new job as co-anchor at WJZ-TV, and I was terrified that I might not measure up. Things weren't working out with my new anchor. He seemed unhappy to have me there.

I lived in the model city of Columbia, Maryland, where all the streets were named after great poets or titles of poems. I lived on Windstream Drive, across the street from the great Columbia Mall. They had some of the best food stalls known to womankind. A whole booth sold nothing but potatoes, any kind you could imagine. And you know I love me some potatoes. They were fried, dipped in vinegar, or baked with cheese and onion.

There was a pizza booth, a corn dog booth, and my favorite at the time, a giant chocolate-chip cookie stall. You could order an 18-inch chocolate-chip cookie with or without macadamia nuts. I loved macadamia nuts. I always ordered the kind with. On weekends I'd stroll the mall, going from stall to stall. Sometimes I'd order something from every booth.

I didn't realize at the time that by overeating, I was trying to fill something deeper, something unconscious. If you had asked me then or even ten years later, I would have answered: "I love chocolate chip cookies." The fact that I was lonely, somewhat depressed, and having a hard time adjusting to the new job never entered my mind.

It was July 1976. I was independent. I had a job most women only dreamed of. I was making my age in salary, with a contract that guaranteed it for three years. I had no reason to be unhappy. But after every six o'clock newscast, I would drive the 30 miles home, always stopping first at the mall. It became a nightly habit.

By the fall of 1976, I had gained ten pounds. I weighed a whopping 148! I went to see my first diet doctor—I still have the check—who put me on a 1,200-calorie eating program and gave me a prescription for diet pills. The pills made me crazy as a betsy bug! I stopped taking them after about a week and tried to cut my 1,200 calories down to 800 to speed up the process. I did lose weight faster, it seemed. In one month I was back to 140, which I decided would be my ideal weight in life. If I only knew then what I know now! Dieting and deprivation only make you gain weight in the long run. It's an endless cycle of deprive, lose, overindulge, gain a little more.

By the end of the year I was 150 pounds. Thus began diet after diet in my search for the perfect weight-loss method. First, the Atkins diet: Eat all the fat, cheese, butter, eggs, and bacon you want, just don't eat any carbohydrates, and be sure to pee on a stick to make sure your body isn't completely breaking down. No one tells you that you're burning muscle as *well as fat, and that's going to make it that much harder to maintain any weight loss. And remember to carry sugarless breath mints. This diet gives you horrible breath.*

In those days, I could lose an average of ten pounds in two weeks. The Scarsdale diet, which allowed some vegetables, was a little better. By the time I went on this one I was up to 160. Then there was the crazy banana, weenie, and egg diet. Didn't they know about cholesterol back then? By Christmas of 1977, I was 165. I no longer considered myself to be just a little overweight. I was beginning to be pained about it. My solution: Go back to the diet doctor and take a weekly aerobics class. This time I tried 1,000 calories a day. Of course I couldn't stick with it. I thought I'd do better with a group. So I joined Weight Watchers, followed by Diet Workshop and Diet Center, and later Nutri-Systems. Every one of these worked—for a while.

In the fall of 1978, I started a talk show called "People Are Talking." Not long after the show began, I interviewed a woman about the revolutionary and fun Beverly Hills diet. This was Atkins in extreme reverse— nothing but carbohydrates. A different kind of fruit each day. Try finding watermelon and kiwi in Baltimore in the middle of winter. After two weeks, I'd lost 10 pounds. In four more weeks I'd gained it back, plus some.

So call me a yo-yo or call me stupid. What would you call someone who keeps doing the same thing, expecting a different result? I continued this pattern throughout my eight years in Baltimore, settling in at 172.

When I heard there was an opening in Chicago for a talk-show host, a lot of people, including me, thought I wouldn't get the job because, first off, I was overweight, and second, I wasn't blond. As a matter of fact, I'll never forget this moment. I was sitting in Dennis Swanson's office—he was the head of ABC's Chicago station, WLS-TV—auditioning for host of the talk show "AM Chicago." ("AM Chicago" later became "The Oprah Winfrey Show.") He was telling me what a gem of a talent he thought I was and how he wanted to hire me right away. I was thrilled, but just in case he hadn't noticed, I wanted to set the record straight. "Well, you know, I'm overweight and black," I declared. "Yeah," he said. "I can see.

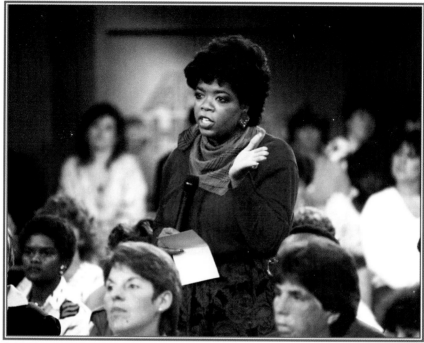

PHOTO BY RICHARD SHAY, © 1985, HARPO PRODUCTIONS, INC.

I'm looking at you. No one in here is going to complain about that." He rubbed his somewhat rounded belly and chuckled. "And as for being black," he continued, "it wouldn't matter to me what color you were. I think you have a gift and I'd like you to share it with this television station."

I was relieved. They weren't going to try to force me to lose weight. It wasn't even a condition for me to be hired. I was home free to eat as I pleased.

When I first moved to Chicago in December 1983, I lived at the Knickerbocker Hotel for a month while looking for a place to call home. Although there was no pressure at all from my bosses to lose a pound or change anything, I thought this could be a new beginning for me, a chance to get motivated and finally get the weight off.

I was so excited about my new job, the city, my staff. Three or four times a week, we'd hit Rush Street, a great Chicago strip lined with restaurants. We'd order margaritas, quesadillas, and cheese nachos. No burgers for me, though; I wanted to keep it "light." So we'd eat "light" cheese nachos and drink light beer and then just split desserts—two to a banana split. I thought I was really doing well by once in a while not rushing out with the staff, opting instead to stay in and order my favorite "light" meal: French onion soup, Caesar salad, and a pasta dish, any one of which could have served as a full meal. If it did not include meat, I thought it was light. I was eating volumes of food.

During those early times, we did one live show a day, so I was done by 10 A.M. At 10:30 we'd start the food search. What would it be today? Taco Bell, Wendy's, Burger King, McDonald's, or the deli. It was a ritual. There were only five of us working on the show. We did everything— booked the guests, made hotel reservations, arranged the limousines, organized the audience. Talking about food—what to eat and where to get it—was our only release. There was only one catch: I was the only one in the group with a weight problem.

In addition to going out for food, there was always something in the office to eat, usually provided by me. I discovered Garrett's popcorn. They pop it while you wait. Cheese, caramel, and plain. I'd get a huge bag of each, vowing to eat the plain and getting the others for my friends at the office. After all, why should they be forced to eat plain? The cheese and caramel mix was just the best!

In one month, I was shocked to find that I weighed 180 pounds. I started feeling more self-conscious. Here I am, a whopping 180, and I was supposed to be losing weight to impress my new Chicago audience. What they must think of me! They obviously think I'm fat.

One day while doing a show with yet another diet expert, I began feeling like a fraud. I just knew everyone else was thinking: Why doesn't she lose weight with her fat butt self. So I thought the best way to handle this is just come clean—stop asking questions like you're some model who doesn't know what a diet is, admit your struggle. So I told the story about the time I'd been trying another diet back in Baltimore.

I had been doing very well, thrown all the snacks out of my house,

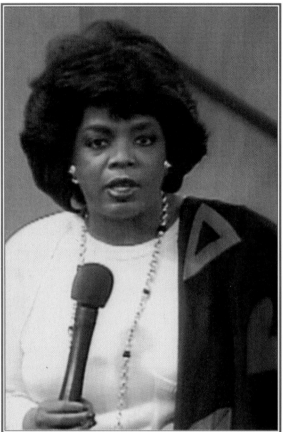

PHOTO BY HARRISON JONES, © 1986, HARPO PRODUCTIONS, INC.

followed all the right diet do's. Then I made the mistake, like a junkie, of visiting my old haunts—the food stalls at the mall. But I didn't succumb to the macadamia-nut cookie or the corn-dog seduction. Instead, I literally ran out of there. I felt that I was being overcome by the smells. After getting home and feeling safe, I was overwhelmed by a compulsion to eat. There was nothing in the house, not even a Rice Krispie! I had made sure of that, determined to succeed this time. As I opened cabinet after cabinet, I found only salt, tabasco sauce, Argo starch, and maple syrup. The fridge was no better, with only baking soda, celery, and a cucumber. And in the freezer,

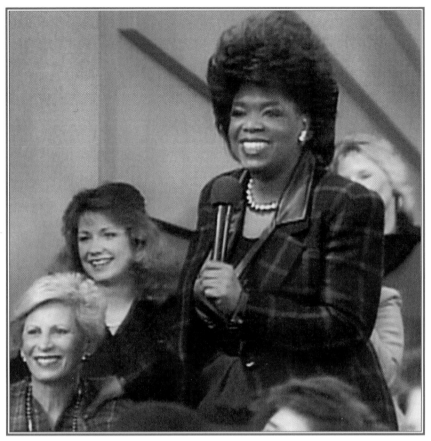

frosted in the corner, solid as a brick, a package of frozen hot-dog buns. Quickly I turned the oven on broil, threw the buns in to thaw out, and even before they could, I grabbed the syrup and smeared it over the partly burnt, partly frozen buns.

Now, looking back, I see no difference between myself and a junkie, scrambling for a needle and whatever dope might be around. Food was my dope.

In that first year of working in Chicago, I had gained 28 pounds. The show started on the first day of January 1984. By December, the first national story had been written about me and the success of the show. The story, called "Chicago's Grand New Oprah," ran in Newsweek magazine. I should have been thrilled at getting national attention. Instead, all I could recall from the story was the writer referring to me as being "nearly 200 pounds of Mississippi-bred black womanhood." "Oh my God," I thought, "do I look nearly 200 pounds?" At that time I was 202, but telling myself I didn't look a pound over 180.

Deep down I knew the truth. Just try shopping when you're over a size 14. Buying clothes was impossible. And when your job is to be on the air every day with a different outfit, it adds to the burden, the guilt, and the frustration of not having anything to wear. So I hired different people to make my clothes. But, I was so ashamed of my size that I would always resist being measured. I didn't want to face the reality of the numbers. I remember a tailor once came to my hotel room in Los Angeles for a fitting. I left him waiting. Finally, I told him he would just have to look at me and guess my size.

The next four years, I would move from 202 to 218, where I stayed for a while. One of my strongest memories is of being at a boxing match where Mike Tyson was fighting Tyrell Biggs. I remember hearing the announcer say, "In this corner, wearing black trunks, weighing 218 pounds, Mike Tyson." He was exactly the same weight I was. I thought, "I weigh as much as the heavyweight champion of the world." I left there determined once again to do something about the weight.

So I hired a trainer. I showed up every day, not because I wanted to be there but because I didn't want to disappoint him. In the process of working out with a trainer for six months, I gained 12 pounds. One day the trainer said, "I think I'm going back to school." I said to him, "So, you're firing me?" He said, "Not exactly, but I think it's better if I go back to school. There are some things I need to work on." That was my first experience with a trainer.

During that four-year period, my goal was to get below 200. No matter what I did, I couldn't. I would get as low as 208 and just stagnate. I'd start a workout program and be inconsistent, fail, and gain more weight.

And I tried every diet program imaginable, including Diets Don't Work. It's like diet therapy done over a weekend. They tell you to eat only when you're hungry, eat exactly what you want, stop when you're full. Then, you try to get to the root of your issues with food. So for two days, I sat in a room with 30 other people, all of us trying to rediscover ourselves. I discovered I needed another approach.

By 1988, I'd had it. I was so depressed and sick of myself. I thought I would try anything short of drugs or stomach stapling. I might have even tried stomach stapling, but I saw a woman who had done it and she had too much skin hanging from her body. I thought, "I don't want a bunch of skin hanging. No, thank you."

Then I heard of Optifast, a fasting and diet supplement program. This was it. This was going to be my savior, my way out. I saw this as the road to freedom.

I saved a pair of Calvin Klein jeans from Baltimore. They were a size ten. They represented a time when I felt better about my body. I thought if I could get to the point where I can get back in those jeans, my whole life would be okay. So that was the goal: Get into the jeans. I saw nothing else but the jeans.

I was an excellent patient. For four solid months, I didn't eat a single morsel of food. I canceled my plans for a vacation in Cap Ferrat, France, and gave the tickets to a friend for a honeymoon present. I realized that there would be no point going to France if I couldn't eat. I canceled all activities that had anything to do with food. And, if I happened to go someplace where there was food, I was unmoved by temptation. After about the third day on the program, I had lost all desire for food. But there were a couple of times in the beginning, I was tempted to eat. That's when I first started to think that maybe something other than being hungry made me want to eat. The only times I was tempted to eat on Optifast were when I felt frustrated or neglected.

I remember coming home one day and Stedman was busy doing something. I kept trying to get his attention but he was obviously interested in whatever he was doing. At that moment, I remember thinking, "I've gotta

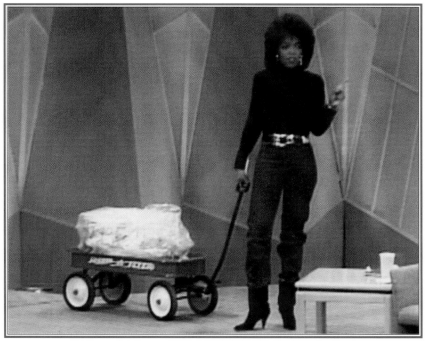

© 1988 HARPO PRODUCTIONS, INC.

eat, I've gotta eat." I later realized what I really wanted was the attention. Another time, I was late at the airport, missed the plane, and had a strong, strong craving for potato chips. Prior to missing the plane, I hadn't been hungry. These were the glimpses that my weight problem was caused not by hunger for food, but by hunger for something else. But I was too out-of-touch with myself to recognize what hunger was.

Instead, I was more interested in watching the pounds come off. I was 211 when I started on Optifast in July 1988. In the first week, I lost 11 pounds. I was ecstatic. In one week, I had already reached the 200 mark. In the first month, I lost 30 pounds. Stedman was away on a business trip in South Africa during that time. He couldn't believe it when he returned. I was 181. I thought my body was getting everything it needed from the packets I was taking. I had no idea that I might be losing muscle weight. Or that my metabolism might be slowing down.

By the fall, I was into the jeans. And proud of it. I was ready to tell the world about how I'd done it. I wanted to share my secret with everyone else who'd struggled. So I went on the air and blew out the Optifast lines that day. Heaven only knows how much money we made for them.

When people would criticize me and say, "Don't worry, she'll put the weight back on," I couldn't imagine what they were talking about. I thought it impossible. Anybody who had shown as much discipline as I had by not eating for four months certainly had licked this problem for good. What I didn't know was that my metabolism was shot. I'd lost muscle weight. I wasn't exercising. And I didn't exercise after losing the weight. There was nothing my body could have done but gain weight.

I weighed 142 pounds when I put on the jeans. It was time to stop taking the supplement and return to real food. I was 142 for one day. The next day I was 145. In two weeks, I was 155. I remember being invited to a party at Don Johnson's house in Aspen and not going because I thought, at 155, I was much too fat for a party with Hollywood types. Oh no, it was starting again. I felt helpless. There was nothing I could do, except pour out my soul in my journal.

November 29th, 1988: Exactly two weeks after the diet show, I've gained five pounds. I'm 150 today. I've been eating out of control. I've got to bring it to an end. I can't get used to being thin.

December 7th, 1988: I read an article today, one criticizing me for the Revlon shoot, making fun of the weight loss, saying, "Let's see her in two years." It really hurt my feelings. I'll show them.

December 12th, 1988: I loved doing the Revlon shoot. It changed the way I felt about me. I never imagined myself as beautiful. But that ad made me feel beautiful. So for that reason alone it was worth shooting just to feel that.

December 13th, 1988: I came home and ate as much cereal as I could hold. I eat junk all day. Not good at all. I've never decided how I'm going to keep the weight off. I keep experimenting, test-

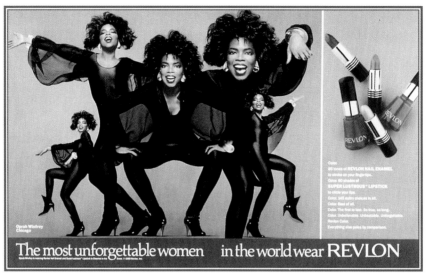

The most unforgettable women in the world wear REVLON

PHOTO BY RICHARD AVEDON FOR REVLON

ing how much I can eat. It's all so ridiculous. How am I going to get through the holidays without gaining?

December 26th, 1988: There's a party in Aspen, I don't want to go. I've gained five more pounds. I'm 155.

January 2nd, 1989: This was my day to start dieting again. Instead, I made pork chops and ate them. Oh, well. Tomorrow's another day, Miss Scarlet. The holidays are officially over. So what's it going to be for me? Fasting again? I don't know if I have it in me.

January 7th, 1989: I'm out of control. Start out my day trying to fast. By noon I was frustrated and hungry just thinking about the agony of it all. I ate three bowls of raisin bran. Left the house and bought some caramel and cheese corn, came back at 3:00 staring at food in the cabinets. And now I want some fries with lots of salt. I'm out of control.

January 19th, 1989: 158 pounds, I'm bordering on disaster. I feel it coming. I'm 158, eating everything in sight. I need help. Old patterns have emerged, are taking over. If I don't fast this entire weekend, then Monday I seek professional counseling. That's the deal, complete and total fast.

January 21st, 1989: I lied to myself about professional counseling. I'm not ready to submit to it.

March 9th, 1989: This is what I wish for, to absolutely eliminate weight as an issue for myself. That I will not eat, drink, or consume anything that will prevent me from reaching my goal. That is what I wish for, the determination and will to do it, just do it no matter what. It is possible and I will.

November 14th, 1989: Anniversary of the diet show, 168 pounds. I'm thoroughly disgusted with myself. I couldn't even get thin for the anniversary show. Where is my resolve? Every day I awaken with good intentions and then I fail.

November 23rd, 1989: Thanksgiving day, 175 pounds, which really is a fat person again. I've lost my resolve trying to find a way to carry on the battle.

December 1st, 1989: I'm still battling what has been for me a lifetime struggle. I thought that after the November 14th–15th diet anniversary show, I could lose weight as an issue. Stop being afraid that someone was going to bring it up and say, "Hey, Oprah, haven't you gained weight?" and go on with my life—not! I'm still struggling. I just cooked rice and smothered chicken for Stedman. I was supposed to eat only a salad. Instead, I ate the salad and the chicken. I'm going to kick this, I just don't know how right now.

December 13th, 1989: The new studio is looking great. We'll be moving in the first of the year. The farmhouse is coming together, too. Everything's going so well, so why I do still feel compelled to eat?

February 16th, 1990: I'm in dire need of help with my weight, almost on the verge of being overcome. I had a woman come and do hair analysis, going to determine what kind of vitamins I need.

It's unbelievable. I'm still looking for a miracle cure. What happened to my New Year's resolution and then my 36-year-old birthday resolution? I don't know. I just know I'm in trouble. I'm 180 pounds. Now I wake every morning hating myself and the weight predicament I'm in. Fifteen pounds ago I would have thought this impossible. I'm not inching, but galloping toward the 200-pound mark. I vow to be back to 150 pounds by the Hope Awards.

April 28th, 1990: I'm exhausted. I worked 20 hours today. Will have to do the same tomorrow. I'm worried about *Brewster Place.* Eating snacks all day from the crafts table. I hate seeing myself on film.

June 12th, 1990: I'm carrying fat around. It's overcoming me, 191 pounds overcome.

June 18th, 1990: I woke up the past four days hating myself because I hadn't fasted or at least stuck to some kind of plan, trying to lose ten pounds in a week so I can put on this suit next week for the Emmys.

July 19th, 1990: Never lost weight for the Emmys. Instead, I gained five more. I'm 196, still trying to reckon myself, still in the closet assessing all the winter clothes I won't be able to wear. Nothing fits. I dread walking into the fat lady's stores. I have nothing to wear to Sally Lu's wedding."

August 11th, 1990: Trying to be in the spirit. The fat has stopped me from feeling; so blocked. I cannot think.

August 15th, 1990: I cried in my office after someone mentioned my clothes and the way I've been dressing: wrong colors, wrong style. Cried because I know that means lots of people have been discussing it. No one says anything. But I feel them avoiding the subject. I cried for my poor miserable self having gotten to this state. Scale said 203 pounds this morning. Controlled—just controlled by it. Every day waking up with a plan. By the end of the day, not following through, feeling diminished, less of a person, guilty, ugly, you name it. Trying to gain control knowing that God says I already have it. Where is it, God? Dancing on the M. C. Hammer show with the fattest behind I've ever seen. I saw that tape and can't deny it anymore. I really am fat again. There in my new fat clothes making me look even bigger, feeling just about as low as one can about myself, knowing that I'm being blocked.

August 25th, 1990: Did a Diets Don't Work seminar. Stood in a room in a bathing suit and admitted that I was 200 pounds. That was hard.

September 9th, 1990: Instead of losing 50 pounds for the Hope Awards, I gained. Had to have the Fabrice gown redone. I didn't want to go; worried about people saying how fat I was. Made the worst-dressed list with Marge Simpson, described as bumpy, dumpy, and down-right lumpy in a gown I thought I looked pretty decent in.

January 29th, 1991: Turned 37. I have a new vision for myself to become lean, fit, strong, physically, emotionally, spiritually. Food alone isn't the answer. What is?

February 20th, 1991: I went on vacation and gained eight pounds, bringing me to an all-time whopping 226 pounds. So big, disproportionate, fat in the face. Unable to move freely, that I don't know this self. My body has betrayed me, or has it just acquiesced? I don't know who this is waddling through the airport. I caught a glimpse of myself reflected in the store window. I didn't recognize the fat lady staring back at me. Stedman says I'm not even close to my potential as a human being, that I let the weight be a barrier. He's right. Sometimes I can feel the connection between my own fears and the weight. So what am I afraid of? That's the question. The answer can set me free.

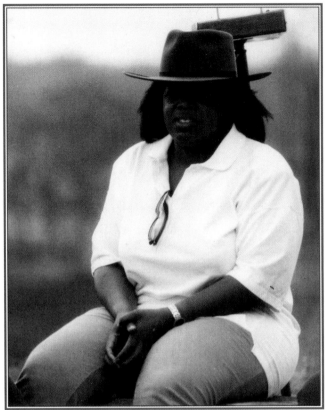

OPRAH WINFREY COLLECTION

My weight consumed my life. There was not a day that passed that I didn't think about it. But I wasn't really doing anything about it. Tomorrow, tomorrow, tomorrow I'm going to stop. I told so many lies to myself about what I was going to do tomorrow. I got tired of hearing my own broken record.

I thought I'd try another trainer. That didn't work. I went to a couple of spas. I lost about four pounds here and there—nothing significant. It was a hard thing to go on the air and say, "I failed. All the people who said I would gain the weight back were right." Then in January 1991, I just gave up. I announced on the cover of People *magazine: "I'll never diet again." When I said that, I didn't mean I was going to give up losing weight. I just* meant that I had to find something that worked. In the meantime, I was going to try to figure out how to be happy with where I was. I thought about those people who say they are fat and happy. Maybe I should try that, just be happy with myself.

Then I decided maybe I just needed to try to be healthier. In August 1991, I visited Cal-a-vie Spa in California. And that's where I met Rosie and talked her into coming to Chicago to be my personal chef. I was weighing in the 220s. With Rosie, everything I ate was low-fat. I also started exercising, just a little, nothing consistent. But at least I was moving. Yet, I continued to gain weight.

But I was feeling no stress, because I was eating it all. Work was becoming more intense, more competitive. More and more talk shows were coming on the market. Knock on wood, we've never lost a season. We've been number one since we started, mainly because we are our number-one competition. Our goal every season is to beat the number from the season before—not our competitors' numbers, but our own. As the market becomes saturated, it takes more effort to do that. But I never really felt the pressure of it all. I had my drug, which was food. I ate my way through children of divorce, abusive husbands, alcoholic mothers, among other show topics. Outwardly, I was becoming more popular and successful. Inside, the burden of weight was always there. It never left me.

I tried not to be depressed about it. Maybe I just needed to accept that I would never be happy with that part of myself. I could achieve career success, but when it came to self-acceptance or discipline, I didn't have it. I did, however, keep searching for it. I couldn't bear to think of myself as a quitter or loser. That's why standing there at the Daytime Emmys at 237 pounds, I decided to try again. I booked three weeks at a new spa in Colorado.

"Okay, so here I am again," I remember thinking, "visiting yet another spa, trying to jump-start myself with another diet. This time I'm going to do it. How many times have I told myself that?" But this time, maybe I would. I was about to meet another trainer who would go through the same routine I'd been through a dozen times.

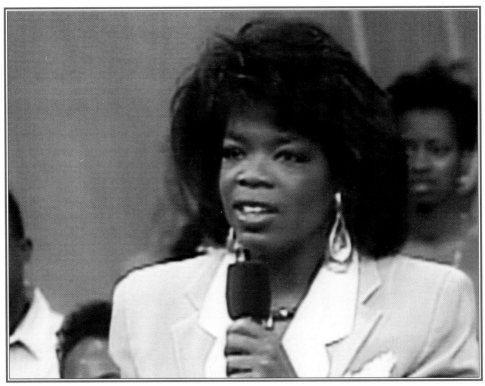

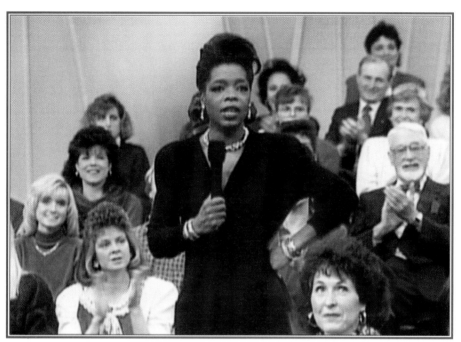

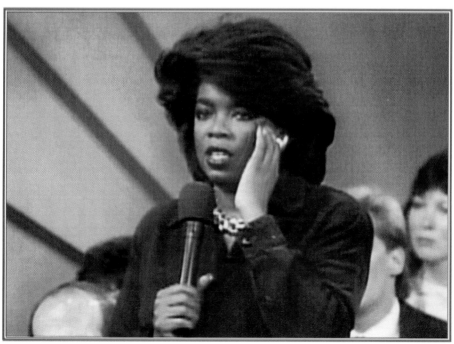

As I was introduced to Bob Greene, I thought, "He must be judging me. He must think, 'What a wallapalooza. I'm supposed to work with her?' " I know if I were him, that's what I would have been thinking. I couldn't look him in the eye.

I no longer had those thoughts after our first hike up Bear Creek. It's a two and a half mile hike winding through the backwoods of Telluride, Colorado, ending at a beautiful waterfall at about 10,000-feet altitude. At the time it was the hardest thing I'd ever done. Bob would say, "Just a little farther." Farther seemed like forever. He encouraged me and made me feel good about what I was able to accomplish.

We hiked every day, lifted some weights, and did either the treadmill or the step machine. I remember standing on the step machine and some petite young missy in a tiny pink polka-dotted outfit stepped on the one next to me. She pushed her level all the way to the top—17 dots. I was panting and holding on for dear life at two dots. I said to myself, "One day, I'm going to be able to blast that machine all the way to the top, too, Missy." And for a moment I had a glimpse that I could.

Often while hiking, Bob and I would talk about why weight was such an issue for me. It was the first time anyone had explained why it had been so easy for me to gain the weight back after fasting. Having a physical explanation for it helped to ease my guilt. Low metabolism, no exercise = weight gain. Volumes of food, even low-fat food = weight gain.

In the three weeks we worked together, I started to lose weight. But Bob didn't want me to weigh in. He wanted my goal to be moving toward a healthier lifestyle and not measuring my life in terms of weight. I started to feel lighter and better about myself.

When I left the spa in Telluride to go to another one in California, I finally weighed myself. I had lost 12 pounds. At the spa in California, I lost another eight pounds. But I had to leave because I twisted my ankle during a hike. I thought this would be a temporary setback. In fact, when I returned to Chicago, weighing 217 pounds, and started the ninth fall season, I found it difficult to exercise consistently with my injured ankle. I made a resolution—like I'd never done that before—to start up full strength, beginning January 1, 1993.

At the beginning of January, I started jogging about three miles a day. I hated every minute of it. I was still eating low-fat, but I was losing no weight. Frustrated, I called Bob.

He came to Chicago, and we had our first workout session on March 15, 1993. I weighed 222 pounds. Bob told me, "I'm only going to work with you if you're willing to be here every day without fail, no excuses. You have to put in at least 40 minutes. And, on a scale from one to ten, you'll need to work at a level seven."

Once again, I so wanted to lose weight. And I really liked Bob's approach. There was nothing bullying or judgmental about it. He was very matter-of-fact and very confident. It was, "If you want to lose weight, this is how you do it." There was no secret. "It's all physics," he said. I believed him. So I looked him straight in the eye and said, "Okay, no problem."

He started walking me at a very vigorous pace. And he modified my eating habits by adding more fruits and vegetables and reducing my portion sizes. The amount of fat in my diet was decreased only slightly, since I was already eating low-fat and had been for two years. I wasn't drinking enough water, though. I've never liked water. But I started drinking lots and lots of it, at least six, sometimes eight, and even ten glasses a day.

The first week, I lost two pounds. Bob had told me that to lose two was a very good thing. I couldn't believe I had worked that hard and lost only two pounds. But two was better than nothing. I was tired at first, doing two shows a day and exercising at a level seven. But I felt good that I had done it for a week, consistently, without fail, no excuses.

The second week, I lost two more pounds. I started to have hope. The third week, I lost an additional pound and really felt good. I got on the scale at the beginning of the fourth week of my program. My heart was shattered. The scale read 223. I followed the plan. I was doing everything right. What went wrong? Bob said, "You're just retaining water, not to worry." Not to worry? I was ready to quit. I'd actually considered taking a packet of some leftover Optifast powder until Bob talked me out of it. It was a low blow holding weight, even if it was water. The following week, I lost the six pounds that had mysteriously appeared the week before, plus two more. Greene was right. I was retaining water. As the weeks went by, that happened every single month. It was a pattern; I could count on it like clockwork. Lose, lose, lose some more, gain, then drop.

We soon switched from walking to jogging, and after a while, I went from jogging three miles to five miles. One day while jogging, Bob said, "I think you should do a race—maybe a ten-K." "I think I will," I said casually. Then later, I thought to myself, "Oh, no, now he's going to expect me to do it."

The next day Bob found races in different parts of the country. There was a 10-K someplace, but there was not enough time to train for it. There was an eight-miler someplace else, but I had other obligations that day. The only race available that I would have time to possibly train for was a half-marathon in San Diego. So I went from "I'm going to run a ten-K" to eight miles, to a half-marathon within an hour's discussion. "What have I gotten myself into? Five months ago I was waddling around the track at 223 pounds," I thought. Bob said, "If you really want to do this, you're going to have to step it up now." The next day, I started running six miles. Within the next couple of weeks, eight miles.

The day of the half-marathon, I was ready. It was so much fun—up until the last mile. People kept saying the end is just around the corner. I had wasted a lot of energy the first eight miles. There's the exhilaration of being with all the runners, and then because everybody knows me in a crowd, I spent the first eight miles waving and smiling. By mile nine, I said, "I need to shut up. I am not going to speak to another person." And so I ran the rest of the race in silence.

I only tired in the last mile. It was straight uphill. I thought it would never end. I knew I wouldn't quit. But I felt the strong possibility my body was going to quit on me. At the finish line, I got a free apple, a cookie, and a T-shirt. I thought, "That's what you get for a half-marathon? Do you get two apples for a whole one?" It was all worth it.

I was as surprised as everyone else that I had done it. It was delightful, this new feeling of accomplishment brought on by pure discipline and self-control. It was exciting. I had always avoided gym class whenever I could. I sat it out or dreaded participating. I never experienced what it felt like to be in control of your body, to train it and have it respond. It was a great feeling. I felt like an athlete. I started paying more attention to every athlete I saw. I'd see pictures of Jackie Joyner-Kersee and go, "Wow, girl, I can relate to what you've been through."

I was so elated over the half-marathon that Bob and I decided to continue to set new goals. I remembered that once while hiking in Telluride I told Bob, "This feels like I'm hiking the Grand Canyon." And Bob said to me, "This is nothing like the Grand Canyon. But you can do that one day." So one day I said to him, "Why not hike the Grand Canyon?" Bob said, "You sure you want to do that?" I told him I ran a half-marathon. I can certainly hike the Grand Canyon.

I remember starting out the hike with my best friend Gayle, Stedman, Bob, and my assistant, Beverly. We were all so excited. We each had about 45 pounds of camp equipment on our backs. We started heading down and I said, "Oh, this will be a piece of cake." That was in the first ten minutes. Four hours later, I was asking for spiritual guidance. Gayle had given up her backpack to me. I thought about that song, "He ain't heavy, he's my brother." Somebody was lying. Because carrying her backpack in addition to mine, it was heavy, sister.

We hiked all the way down. It took us five and a half hours. We spent the night in the bottom of the Canyon, and hiked out the next day. Going up was twice as hard. I was proud to have accomplished it. But next time, I'll buy a postcard. Because let me tell you, the Canyon looks exactly the way it does on the postcard. It's no different. Those postcards are really good.

By November 1993, I was goal weight: 150 pounds. I even got down as low as 148 while running eight-minute miles. I can't tell you what a feeling of accomplishment I had by reaching that weight. I had fulfilled my goal of wanting to be strong and lean and fit and healthy. And I did it the right way. I literally never felt better. Normally in the old days I would have

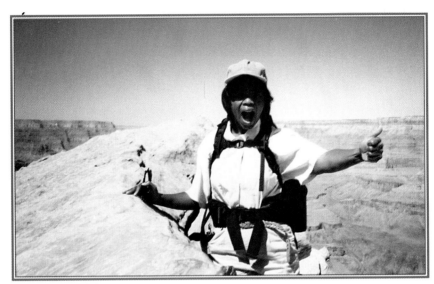

OPRAH WINFREY COLLECTION

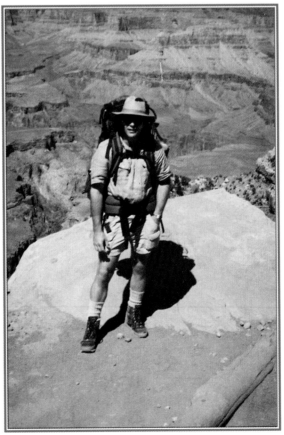

OPRAH WINFREY COLLECTION

wanted to celebrate by going out and eating a good meal. But because so much of my life was changing with the discipline it took to get up and work out every day, I wanted to celebrate my 40th year, not with just champagne toasts but with something that would be symbolic of my health and strength. I decided I would run a full marathon.

At the time I made the decision to do it, I was running about five miles a day. I knew that my mileage would have to increase. Bob said, "It's going to require a lot of you. Are you sure you can devote the time, given your schedule? Can you train and do two shows a day?" I said, "No problem."

"No problem" really meant having to rearrange my schedule depending on where I was. That meant sometimes getting up at 4:30 in the morning and running almost every day, no matter what. I remember one day it was pouring rain, and I said to Bob, "Well, can't run today." He said, "Why not?" And I said, "Because my hair will get wet." And he said, "So what, your hair will get wet." I told him, "You know how us black women are about our hair. We can't get our hair wet." He said, "That's nonsense. I'm afraid you will have to get your hair wet. If it's any consolation, mine'll get wet too." I pleaded, "You don't understand. It's a cultural thing."

He dragged me out. I complained every step of that 12-mile run up Lake Shore Drive. It poured. I was soaked. My hair got soaked. It was the weekend and Andre had the day off. But I managed to dry my hair and make do.

What makes training for a marathon difficult is you have to get the training in no matter what else is going on in your life. And I have a whole other complete, full life. I have the show, and the show must go on. I would do ten or 12 miles in the mornings before shows. I'd save the long runs, 15 to 20 miles, for the weekends.

I remember the first time I ran 12 miles. I could always determine when I reached 12, because that's when my legs would start turning to stone. My left leg always felt like a cement block. I'd think, "Oh this must be the twelfth mile, I can feel that little cement block coming on." As I got

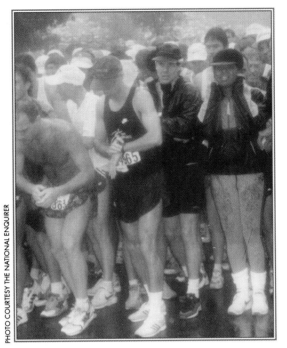

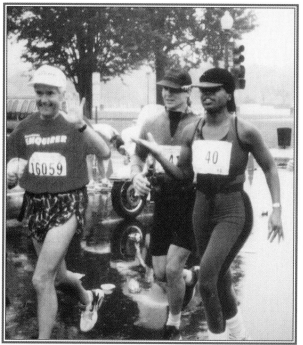

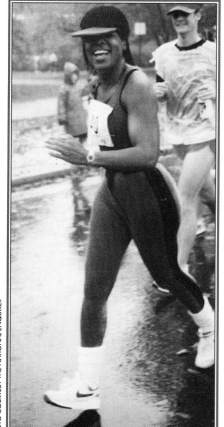

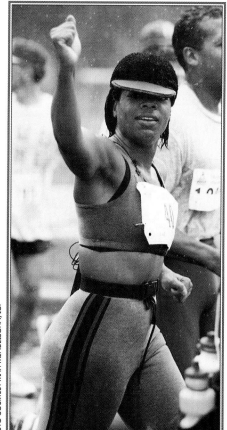

stronger, I wouldn't feel it until the 18th mile. The first day I ran 18 miles, I was in awe of myself. After the run, I got in the car and went out and drove it. I could not believe it. Eighteen miles is a long way.

We usually ran on the road, single file, with Bob running slightly ahead. I never ran with earphones. I'd sing to myself, meditate, ask myself, "What the hell am I doing out here?" There were moments when it became surreal and moments when I felt really good that I had the strength to just do it. I felt like a Nike ad.

Well, the big day arrived. And wouldn't you know it, it was pouring rain—a damp, cold rain. And, yes, I was ready for it. I'd been soaked a few times before. It rained the entire four and a half hours that I ran. By the fifth mile, my jacket was so soaked, I took it off and threw it away. It was weighing me down.

I never even felt the first three miles. A lot of runners make the mistake of running too fast in the beginning of the race. They get caught up in all the excitement. This started to happen to me, then Bob said, "You've got to slow down a little." My goal was to run about nine-minute miles and I just ran the first three in under 24 minutes. I made the adjustment.

I was wearing the number 40 for my age. I forced myself to drink water every three miles, whether I wanted it or not. I was focused and determined. I spoke to almost no one. When people would shout out my name, I would just nod or raise a hand. We passed monuments and parks and cheering crowds and even a marching band or two. I never looked up. Focused.

The National Enquirer had hired two of their guys to follow me. It's the first time I ever talked to a tabloid reporter. They became my checkpoint buddies. "How far away are we, guys?" They'd say, "Oprah, you're at mile nineteen. Keep going, you look great."

Around the 21st mile, I got that old concrete feeling. But at 21, with only five to go, there wasn't a chance I'd stop. When I saw I only had one mile to go, I was overwhelmed with feelings that are to this day difficult to explain.

Flashing through my mind was every year of this weight struggle: every

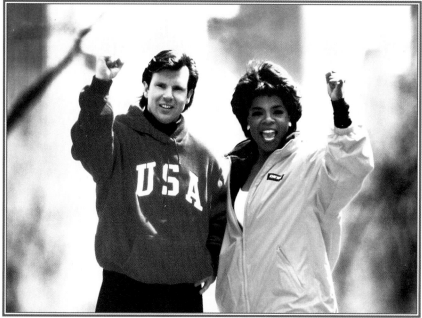

time I prayed to get rid of the weight, every time I tried another diet, every time I'd failed, every time I wanted to be in control of my body and my life but couldn't find the means to do it. Every bad meal, every stuffed feeling, every repressed emotion, I was feeling now. I was overcome with exhilaration for what I had done. I could see the finish line. I could actually see the finish line.

Running a marathon is a metaphor for life, I think. It has its obstacles, moments when you feel like giving up, when you're tired, overwhelmed. But you keep going. Finally, you can see the finish line. The purpose is clear.

It was a proud and joyful moment, one of the best I've ever had.

Since that time, it's been hard to maintain running at that level. So I picked up some weight several months after the marathon. I still work out every day, though not as hard. When you're not willing to work as hard and you have a set-point like mine, you gain weight—sometimes more than you would like. For a brief time I was up as much as 17 pounds. I try to stay in the low to mid 150s. 150 is best for me, but to stay there, I have to work incredibly hard. With my current schedule that's not always possible. And that's okay, I've accepted that.

All of the information about exercise, eating right, and how my body works helped me change the physical me. The most important part is to understand that it's not as much about the weight as it is about making the connection. That means looking after yourself every day and putting forth your best effort to love yourself enough to do what's best for you. I have to say that's the greatest gift Bob Greene has given me. The biggest change I've made is a spiritual one. It comes from the realization that taking care of my body and my health is really one of the greatest kinds of love I can give myself. Every day I put forth the effort to take care of myself. And there's no question I'm living a better life.

—**Oprah Winfrey**

We don't see things as they are,
we see them as we are.
–Anais Nin

IT was the summer of 1992, and I was about to meet Oprah Winfrey. At the time, I was the fitness director for a new spa in Telluride, Colorado, and Oprah was one of our first guests. I wondered if I was the only person in America who had never seen "The Oprah Winfrey Show." But I certainly knew who she was. As I sat in my office waiting to meet her, I thought about the first time I had heard her name.

It was back in 1987, and I was in charge of a health and fitness program at a South Florida hospital. There was one particular week when we were flooded with calls about one of our weight-loss classes. The reason for this sudden interest, I soon found out, was Oprah's first significant weight loss and the show she did about it. She began that show by pulling out a wagon loaded with 67 pounds of fat to dramatize how much weight she'd lost. She had dropped the pounds by using the Optifast fasting and supplement system.

I was quite familiar with such diets, since we offered one at the hospital. But I firmly believed that a fasting and supplement program should be used as a last resort, and then only for a few select individuals—certainly not the average person trying to lose weight. These diets have many risks, including gall-bladder complications, heart palpitations, and feelings of depression, and the resulting weight loss is almost always temporary. I knew someone as popular as Oprah Winfrey could inspire a lot of imitators, and I didn't have a good feeling

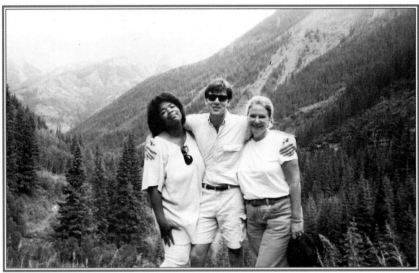

OPRAH WINFREY COLLECTION

about it. I also didn't think Oprah could keep the weight off once she stopped taking the supplement and began eating real food again.

My instinct was confirmed the following year when she regained all the weight she lost, plus some. That story also made national news, and the hospital again received a large increase in calls. I was amazed that one individual could have such a tremendous impact on our industry. Yet, I felt bad for her, as I would for anyone who struggles with a weight problem. I find it hard to believe, but I remember daydreaming at the time that I would like to meet her. I thought, "I could really help her."

Now, two years later, here I was about to meet her. Shortly after leaving the hospital, I had moved to Colorado to help open the Doral Telluride Resort and Spa. It was an unusual move for me, leaving a prestigious position and accepting less money than I was used to, but I was drawn there. I had always wanted to live, work, and ski in a beautiful western mountain town. I had even considered working as a ski instructor after graduate school, but I knew it was probably time to grow up and use my degree.

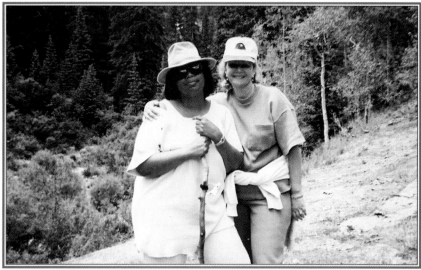

OPRAH WINFREY COLLECTION

As an exercise physiologist, I had worked in medical settings for about a decade, helping people lose weight and drastically change their lifestyle for health or medical reasons. In recent years, I found that most of my time was spent with administrative duties, personnel headaches, and paperwork. I really missed working one-on-one with clients.

When the spa opened, and I was asked to work with Oprah, I didn't hesitate. As I sat in my office pondering how all these seemingly coincidental events in my life had led up to the moment I once daydreamed about, I heard voices in the corridor. Someone was being given a tour. It was Oprah. I left my office to meet her.

When I was introduced to Oprah, I looked her directly in the eyes, as I always try to do when I speak to someone. "It's a pleasure to meet you," I said. But I couldn't help noticing how she quickly averted her eyes and looked straight down at the floor. I later thought, "Did I stare too directly? Is it a celebrity thing? Does she not want to be here?" Then it dawned on me that this was the same reaction I get virtually every time I meet new clients who want to lose weight.

The feeling of embarrassment about their predicament is so great that they often avoid looking me in the eye. Moreover, they expect that I am passing judgment on them for being overweight, much like they do themselves. I guess I didn't expect such a reaction from Oprah Winfrey, who is the star of her own television show, and the winner of multiple Emmy awards, not to mention a worldwide icon. She was noticeably uncomfortable. But she had no reason to be. The truth is, especially at that moment, I had tremendous respect for her, as I do for anyone attempting the challenge of permanent weight loss.

Over long hikes and workouts, Oprah and I laughed, shared stories, and generally grew comfortable with each other. One day we were hiking along with her good friend Arleen and, in an attempt to learn something about me, Oprah asked, "So, Bob, where are you from?" I told her I grew up in New Jersey. "Oh, that's near Stedman," she said. I thought maybe she was confused. "No, you must mean Camden," I responded. "I don't know of a Stedman, New Jersey." Suddenly, Oprah broke up with laughter, but for the life of me I couldn't figure out why. Finally, when she was able to compose herself, she explained to me that Stedman was the first name of her boyfriend, Stedman Graham. She was simply bemused that she had met someone so unaware of her very public life. Arleen gave me a look like "You've been living up in these mountains too long." I got the feeling that Oprah liked the fact that I knew so little about her life and that I didn't even own a television.

(I now know Stedman Graham quite well, and I have to say he was very supportive of Oprah during the difficult process of shedding the weight. So often, the important people in your life act to sabotage your efforts, usually in very subtle ways. This subtle sabotage is usually not malicious or even intentional, but can undermine even the most committed person.)

During her three-week spa visit, Oprah and I hiked many miles in the San Juan mountains and spent a lot of time in the gym. I figured she had lost about ten pounds, but I didn't want her to weigh herself, because I knew she would be disappointed if the scale didn't reflect a large weight loss. Oprah is a person who expects a lot of herself— perhaps too much. I'll never forget how after one week of training she said she wanted to run a marathon by the time she was 40. I knew that she was going to be 39 that January and that she weighed approximately 233 pounds, and that she tapes two, sometimes three shows a day in addition to running her company. Most anyone would have thought she was just making idle conversation, but I took her seriously. I knew she could do it.

By the end of her stay, Oprah had lost between 10 and 12 pounds. Both she and I were thrilled with the results. I felt confident of her commitment to lose the weight, but I also recognized the enormous task she had ahead of her to permanently change her life. As we parted, she said, "You wait, I'll be back this fall and I'll be cute as a button." I smiled and thought, what a fun three weeks.

Meeting Oprah, I learned four very important things about her:

- She was physically capable of exercising at the proper intensity levels.

- She basically knew how to eat healthy.

- She possessed the will and desire to make the changes in her life that would result in permanent weight loss.

- She was either unaware of, or greatly underestimated, the depth and complexity of the emotional issues that contributed to her being overweight.

Oprah is a source of inspiration in so many ways. She has been blessed with so many gifts, but a favorable metabolism is not one of them. In addition, for most of her life, she has used food to cope with stressful or painful events. These are the reasons she is such a great role model for people attempting to permanently change their lives. For Oprah to maintain her weight at the level she desires, she must work extremely hard—much harder than the average person. She also must find healthier ways to deal with life's problems—in a life that sees problems on a daily basis. This is not to say that she always follows my program to the letter, but she realizes that when she does, she gets results quickly, and when she doesn't, it is her choice. She also knows that this new, healthier way of eating, living, and thinking has greatly improved the quality of her life. She now has control over her life, and you can too!

I have outlined ten steps I believe are the fastest and healthiest way to increase your metabolism and shed excess weight. When performed daily, the ten steps are the most effective way to lose pounds and stay healthy. There are no shortcuts. This is not a book with quick fixes and easy answers. You will gradually progress within your ability, but it will require you to work hard each day. However, if you follow all ten steps consistently, you *will* see results! First, there are some basics you need to learn before undertaking the program. More important, you need to determine if you're even ready to make the commitment to having a better body—and a better life.

—**Bob Greene**

Why We Eat

IN a perfect world, we would eat simply for the sheer pleasure of experiencing different foods. Or we might eat for the enjoyment of the company with whom we share our food. But as you know, the world is not perfect. There are many reasons why we eat. Some reasons we are aware of, and some we may not be.

FOOD AS NUTRITION

Fulfilling its most basic purpose, food provides us with energy. This energy is carried within the molecules of three basic nutrients: carbohydrates, fats, and protein. These three nutrients are referred to as macronutrients. When our bodies break them down, energy is released. This energy is used for all our basic body functions, as well as for exercise. Excess energy is stored as fat for later use.

Aside from providing energy, food gives us water and essential vitamins and minerals, called micronutrients. We need all of these to sustain life. Vitamins are organic substances needed for almost all body processes. Minerals are metallic elements essential for a process called metabolism. Water is a truly amazing nutrient. It's involved in virtually all of the body's many functions. We can receive water by drinking it and by extracting it from the foods we eat. We need water daily.

This brief introduction to nutrition gives you reasons why we *must* eat. Certainly, we can also *choose* to eat.

FOOD FOR PLEASURE

Let's face it, for most of us food is a true pleasure. And eating should be a pleasure, one to be enjoyed and experienced. With so many restaurants, cookbooks, food magazines, gourmet food stores, even a cable cooking channel, we have taken the art of eating to new heights—and the art of cooking, as well.

There is so much for us to appreciate about food: its taste, its smell, its texture, how it looks. It can remind us that we are alive. In this way, food is miraculous. And we can enjoy it alone or with others.

Social Eating

Food has always been part of social functions, and will always remain so. It's an essential part of family traditions, whether for special occasions or daily meals. You know how it's sometimes impossible to visit family without eating something? They can be offended if you refuse.

Food is also an important part of friends getting together. What would a Friday night date be without dinner and a movie? Can you imagine what a card game would be like without food? It's the central focus for many types of celebrations. What's a holiday without food? What would we do at weddings? Food is part of our culture. But when we begin to use food to excess and eat for reasons other than nutrition and enjoyment, we often run into problems.

USING FOOD TO DEAL WITH STRESS

Working as closely as I do with Oprah, I have had a lot of time to observe her eating habits. It didn't take me long to figure out when and why she ate. I was watching her one evening as she paced up and down the carpet in her office. Each time she would pass the coffee table, she would pluck some grapes. She would then turn and walk toward an end table and reach for a handful of popcorn. After a few minutes of watching this, I asked her, "Had a rough day?" She stopped and said, "How'd you know?" I replied, "Well, it's obvious. You've just had three handfuls of snacks, and I've only been here four minutes!" She put the grapes back on the table and sighed. I could tell it had just dawned on her that she was eating not because she was hungry, but because she was stressed. This often unconscious eating due to stress is all too common. I'm sure at some time or another, it has happened to all of us.

The baby is screaming, you're rushing to get the older kids off to school, you burn your hand on the toaster, and the phone rings: The baby-sitter can't make it. When the chaos cools down, you go to the refrigerator and eat the last half of the Boston cream pie you were saving for the family's dessert that evening. Or you're at your desk at work, an important report is due, the client who was upset with you last week is on the phone requesting a meeting, and your boss pops in every ten minutes to see where that report is. You remember that candy bar in your top drawer.

Taking pleasure in food, eating socially, even using food to deal with stress are behaviors we all can identify with. They are common and socially acceptable, and we even joke about them. But when we use any of them too often, a weight problem can develop. For some of you, one or a combination of these behaviors is the primary cause of your weight problem.

Your road to a healthier lifestyle will be considerably easier than someone who has deeper emotional issues. Your weight loss, however, might be complicated by daily circumstances—circumstances that need to be recognized, examined, and remedied. Not too long ago, I worked with a stock trader named Louise. During our exercise sessions, Louise would describe what it was like in the "pit," or the trading floor. It sounded tremendously stressful.

Her exercise sessions were great, but she couldn't seem to lose those last 12 pounds. I knew this was related to her eating habits, which were in turn related to her stressful job. It wasn't until she started keeping a journal, switched her exercise time to the morning, began bringing her own food to work, and found an appropriate outlet for her stress—taking a walk—that she was able to shed the last 12 pounds. Louise did not have any significant emotional issues that contributed to her being overweight. It was her lifestyle that led to the excess pounds. She needed to find another way besides eating to deal with stress in her life.

Like Louise, you may be greatly challenged in your weight loss by extreme stress in your work or home life. For you it's important to not only exercise and eat right, but also to become more aware of when and why you eat. Keeping a journal at the beginning of your program will be helpful in recognizing what causes you stress as well as when you are most likely to be stressed and, therefore, abuse food. You can record instances when you use food to get you through stressful situations or overuse food in social settings. You can also write down what you were thinking and feeling at the time. This can help you uncover the reasons you overeat. I'll talk more about keeping a journal in Step Ten.

I know it's difficult to change your habits—and, ultimately, your life. But you can do it. If you follow the steps outlined in this book, with a little discipline, effort, and willpower, you will attain your weight-loss goals and gain self-control.

But if you have deeper emotional issues, the weight-loss process becomes more complicated.

THE EMOTIONAL SIDE OF EATING

I had been working with Oprah for about three months when I noticed that almost every week she would go out with her friends to

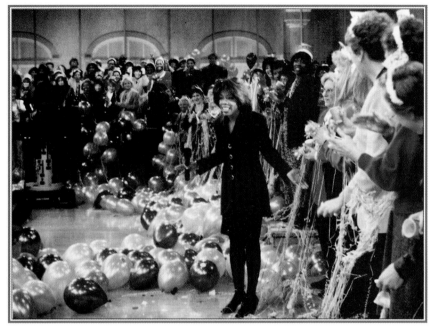

HARPO ENTERTAINMENT GROUP

celebrate some special event—a birthday, anniversary, holiday, even a good show. During these get-togethers, she would always eat something that wasn't very healthy for her. I wasn't overly concerned because she was following the program otherwise, and, as I said earlier, eating is a normal social activity. But I knew it was important to find out why she was straying so frequently. Once, after she had come back from some such event, I confronted her: "You're doing so well most of the time. Why do you eat so poorly when you go out with your friends?"

Her initial response was, "What do you mean? I'm not supposed to celebrate the show's eighth anniversary? It was only some fried calamari." I pointed out to her that she was celebrating something every week, and, more important, she was eating what she knew she shouldn't. Then, as Oprah described her nights out, it occurred to me that each time she got together with her friends, she felt pressured to eat and drink with them. They were making suggestions like, "Hey, we're celebrating, can't you just have a little of this?" and "You mean you can't have just one glass of wine (which would turn into two or three)?" I knew it was a problem that some of her friends weren't supporting her commitment to lose weight, a problem that would have to be dealt with. But there was also a more basic problem.

I told Oprah, "What I think is going on is that you just don't want to let your friends down." She was silent for a moment. Then she said, "I've had this problem since childhood." I knew for her to admit this to me was a breakthrough. Oprah's need to please people by never saying no extended from events in her childhood. She thought if she said no, her friends wouldn't like her anymore. This may sound simplistic. But it was the reason she wouldn't refuse an invitation to eat with her friends, even though she knew it was undermining her efforts to lose weight.

She not only lacked the will to say no, but going out to a restaurant played right into another problem she had. Food was Oprah's primary coping mechanism. She sought refuge in food whenever she felt unloved or bad about herself. Eating made her feel comforted and safe—even loved. So, she literally buried her problems under food. She ate to cushion herself from bad news and bad feelings. Food became a narcotic. It buffered her from pain, sadness, anxiety, any emotion she did not want to feel.

The fact that her friends were tempting her is a whole separate issue that I will talk about later in the chapter. But the main point here is to illustrate how deeply rooted emotional issues can control your eating habits.

We all have different ways of coping with pain. Some people use alcohol and drugs, others immerse themselves in their work, some take it out on others, and still others use food. Food just happens to be the most socially acceptable coping mechanism. It's also the most physically evident. With food, you're very often wearing your pain.

Yet I would guess that most of us at some point in our lives have used food to cope with life's problems. How much and how often you do this can help you determine the extent to which your emotional issues contribute to your weight problem.

The kind of emotional issues I'm referring to generally come from childhood experiences or traumatic events. They can influence everything from your eating and exercise habits to your self-perception. If eating is your primary way of coping with these issues, you'll have a much longer, more complicated, and sometimes even painful journey ahead of you in order to achieve permanent weight loss. It will also be incredibly rewarding if you are successful.

Oprah clearly used food as her primary coping mechanism. For her, being overweight was both a physical and an emotional problem. And in order to make permanent changes in her life, Oprah had to deal with the underlying emotional issues she had been avoiding with food.

We may not even be aware of what our emotional issues are. Such is the case with 36-year-old Barbara. Before I agree to work with new weight-loss clients, I always have at least a two-hour consultation with them. During such a consultation with Barbara, I learned that at least two or three times a week, she would eat uncontrollably and have feelings of great depression afterward. She displayed a common and classic eating disorder. What was not clear to her was why she had these episodes. I asked her if she was receiving professional counseling, and she was. I decided that I could help her with an exercise and eating plan.

During our twice-weekly exercise sessions, she would often tell me funny stories about her dating encounters. I recalled from the consultation that she began binge-eating at age 22. On a hunch, I asked her if she was dating back then. She said she'd had a bad breakup with a guy about six months before these eating episodes appeared. Bingo.

The amazing thing is that at first, Barbara was uncertain whether the two events were related. With the help of another therapist, she was able to understand the impact her emotional issues regarding men had on her eating. She was able to stop bingeing and reach her goal weight.

Again, when you eat for reasons other than hunger, it is helpful to write down what you ate, how much you ate, and why you ate. Your feelings when you started and when you stopped eating are important to note as well. Your journal can be a valuable tool.

If emotional issues are tied to your eating habits, the steps in this book are extremely important to learn and follow, but additional support is almost always needed. This support can come from a professional counselor, a supportive friend or relative, a dietitian, or an exercise specialist—and in many instances, all of the above. The type and amount of additional support will vary, depending on the complexity of the emotional issues. Your primary physician can also point you in the right direction and should be consulted before you undertake any new program.

You will find that as you become more fit, you will become more aware of what you feel. In addition, food will be less of a buffer to your stress or emotional pain. This happened for Oprah. I remember she had dropped 70 pounds and was eating healthy and exercising regularly when she experienced her first headache. I mean her first headache ever! We were running around an indoor track and she wasn't her usual cheerful self, so I asked her if something was wrong. "I have a headache," she said. "Do you get those often?" I persisted. "No, I've never had one before," she replied. Of course, I didn't believe her, and proceeded to ask her three more times. "You mean you've never had a headache?" Her response was no every time.

In the past, Oprah would simply go to the refrigerator and eat the stress or pain away. But when she no longer used eating as an outlet, she began to experience physical pain. Pain is a part of life. I'm happy to report Oprah now also experiences backaches, muscle spasms, and cramps!

Oprah now experiences her emotional pain as well, instead of burying it under food. And because she deals with it in a healthy way, she was able take off her excess weight and keep it off.

Keeping the weight off is actually the greatest challenge of this process. Just look at the statistics on long-term weight loss and you'll understand how difficult the journey can be for anyone attempting it: About 95 percent of all people who begin a weight-loss program regain the pounds within five years. Not a comforting statistic!

But I know you can beat those odds. In studying the relatively few people who are successful, I have found that they always go through two stages in their weight loss. Both stages are important for anyone attempting permanent weight loss. The first stage is to adopt healthy eating and exercise habits that become a natural part of your lifestyle. Describing and implementing these lifestyle changes will be a primary focus of this book. The second stage requires you to make what I call "the connection."

THE CONNECTION

I was in the middle of an initial consultation with Sandra. As she ran down the list of all the unsuccessful diets and weight-loss programs she had done over the past ten years, her husband poked his head in to say hello. They both seemed very nice; I liked them immediately.

Sandra wanted to lose about 30 pounds, a very realistic goal. During the consultation, I modified Sandra's diet, but not all that much since she already had a good idea of how to eat properly. She was already exercising, but I needed to make a few changes there as well. After about six weeks, Sandra had lost just four pounds and was quite disappointed. But then again, she never seemed overly happy about her accomplishments. I explained to her that four pounds was fine, and that it may be a slow process. What's more important, I told her, is the way you feel. After our talk, she felt much better. Then, during our next workout together, she admitted her eating and exercising had both suffered. She also mentioned she'd had an argument with her husband and that they hadn't spoken all week.

In the months that followed, Sandra would tell me more and more about her home life. It was clear that while she cared very much about John, her husband, there were serious problems. Her weight had hit a plateau, although it was down almost 20 pounds from when I first started working with her. She wanted to be at her goal weight more than anything. I sensed that the cause of her plateau was her unhappiness with her marriage. It caused her to eat when she shouldn't. I also knew that being married was extremely important to her, and she was afraid to make significant changes in her life. When she asked me what she would need to do to break through her plateau, I told her she needed to look at her entire life and make herself happy.

It was approaching summer, and I had to tell Sandra I would be traveling for six weeks with Oprah. I told her that we could resume our workouts together once I got back in town, but I didn't think she needed my help anymore. For a moment she looked lost, then said, "You're right."

When I returned, I checked on all my past and present clients, including Sandra. She had great news: She had reached her goal weight, her career had taken off, and, in her words, "My life is wonderful." This did not sound like the same person. "Oh yeah," she added, "John moved out." I asked her, "Wasn't it difficult?" Her reply was: "Yes, very. It's the best thing for both of us and I'm at the point now where I'm doing what's best for me. I care too much about myself."

Those were the magic words. Sandra made what I call "the connection." And her life changed forever. It is rarely as easy as it was for Sandra, but it can be done.

The connection is a change in perception. It is first realizing that losing weight is not what is most important. Instead, the excess weight is merely a symptom of a larger problem and losing it is a side effect, a nice one certainly, of something much more important. It is really about increasing self-confidence, inner strength, and discipline. It is about feeling better on a daily basis, having control over your life, and caring about yourself. Ultimately it is about self-love.

The connection rarely happens immediately. It is more likely to occur as you experience weight loss and the corresponding positive life-changes. As your weight improves, so does your life, and vice versa. That's because your weight, your self-image, and even your body reflect other things in your life.

You can create a positive cycle in your life. As you begin to lose weight, you will start this positive cycle of feeling better about yourself, which will help motivate you to continue your new lifestyle, which in turn will cause you to shed more excess pounds and again feel even better about yourself. As you approach your ideal body weight, you will be in a better mental position to make the connection, because you will be caring even more about yourself. You will want only the best for you, which means exercising and eating right, as well as dealing with your problems in a healthy way. You will know you've made the connection when you care enough about yourself that you don't consider doing anything outside your best interest.

Fully making the connection will happen only when you are ready. It will require you to make many changes, both in your perception and your actions. You cannot force it. But knowing it can occur is all that is needed at this time. Again, a primary purpose of this book is to start you on the first stage of the journey—the physical steps, or healthy eating and exercise habits involved in shedding pounds and maintaining your ideal body weight. Another important purpose of this book is to introduce you to the possibility that the way you feel about yourself dictates much of your behavior and can influence how you treat yourself. And how you treat yourself on a daily basis has a tremendous effect on your physical appearance. To complete the cycle, your physical appearance affects how you feel about yourself. This cycle can move in either a positive or negative direction.

Oprah has put into motion the positive cycle of improving her weight and her life. Because she now cares more about herself, she treats herself better each day, she cares for and protects herself, and she is also able to confront her friends about undermining her weight-loss efforts and actually get their support. Now, she no longer uses the need to please her friends as an excuse to overeat.

Many of Oprah's friends also had to adjust to her new way of life. This will probably happen to you and your loved ones, as well.

WHEN FRIENDS AND LOVED ONES DON'T SUPPORT OUR EFFORTS

I have never worked with anyone wishing to lose weight who was not adversely affected by someone close to them. I have been in this field for 15 years and this still amazes me. The degree to which this is a problem varies considerably, but it almost always exists and you should be conscious of it. This form of sabotage can be obvious or subtle. The person carrying it out may not even be aware of it. And the reasons for it are as varied as people are.

What it always comes down to is how your impending weight loss is going to affect the person doing the sabotage. Some of Oprah's friends were clearly threatened by her losing weight, perhaps because they feared she might not have as much in common with them. Perhaps they thought she would choose not to spend as much time with them. Perhaps her weight loss would even affect how she felt about them. Ultimately, it could lead to their losing her friendship. Nothing could be farther from the truth, but we are not always rational beings.

This was not the extent of Oprah's battles with those she cared about. Many of Oprah's fans also felt she was leaving them behind by losing the weight. This bothered her, but not enough to go off her program. In years past, this issue could have caused her to abandon her weight-loss efforts, since she still had such a strong need to please

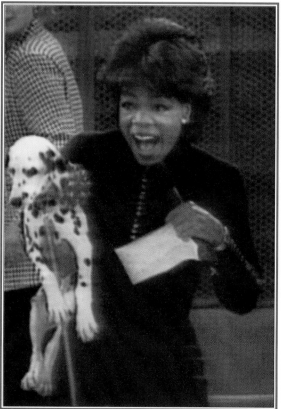

people. Instead, Oprah decided to do a show about it. One woman on the show admitted that, although she once dreamed of having Oprah over for dinner, now that Oprah had lost weight, this woman was unsure whether she even wanted Oprah to drop by.

Don't underestimate how people are affected by your weight loss. Often the more weight you lose, the more this problem is magnified. Just see what happens when you make the connection. As Sandra got closer to her goal weight, her husband's fears became greater. He worried they would have less in common, that she might leave him. He went so far as to create obstacles to not only her weight loss but her professional goals as well. He wasn't doing it maliciously. In fact, he wasn't even aware of what he was doing. But she had to find the strength to stand up for what she really wanted in order to achieve her goals. Yes, she lost her marriage, but she gained her self-respect and much more.

When you make the connection, your life will change. And there may be people close to you who don't want it to change. If your friends and family don't give you the support you need, losing weight can be an uphill battle. My advice to you before undertaking this program is to try to bring those people on board as early as possible. Have them read this book or at least this section. Let them know you're doing more than just a weight-loss or fitness program; you are transforming your life. Ask them for their support. They may even want to participate in your new way of life.

Lack of support from those around you can be a roadblock in the journey to change your life. There may be others. The physical steps involved in making that journey will soon be discussed, but your ultimate success depends on creating a sound mental foundation, starting with being self-aware.

Becoming Self-Aware

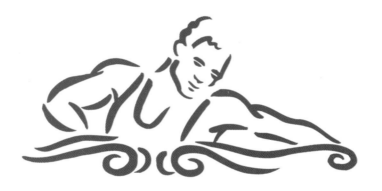

ONLY when you have self-awareness can you achieve self-acceptance. Only when you accept yourself can you experience self-love. And when you are capable of self-love, you learn to love. To express love is our ultimate goal. And you thought you'd bought a weight-loss book! You did. But this is the path that leads you to the connection. And making the connection will change your life.

I know you are eager to begin the steps. But before you can make any physical changes, you need to know yourself. This is the foundation that will help you transform your life. Think of what happens when you build a house on a shaky foundation. It eventually crumbles. This is one of the reasons that so few individuals maintain their weight loss. If you don't know who you are or what you want, or you are unhappy with yourself, or you believe losing weight is the answer to all your problems, I can almost guarantee that the weight you lose will come back.

We all need to accept and love ourselves, no matter how we look. That means loving ourselves just as much now as when we reach our goal. Remember that food can be used as an anesthetic for dulling pain, but the original problem that caused you pain may remain unresolved. Not facing your problems now or along the way to your goal weight will only make it easier for you to lapse back into your old habits for dealing with pain.

Whether or not food is your primary way of dealing with pain, you can benefit from this chapter. This chapter helps set the stage for making the connection. Becoming self-aware can be a difficult process. If any of you find that confronting these issues causes you great distress, I recommend you see a professional counselor for additional support. Losing weight alone can't transform your life. Changing your perception can.

GETTING TO KNOW YOURSELF

Chances are, you're reading this book to help you change some aspect of your life. You are probably looking to make physical changes. Understand that this will require you to make changes in your behavior—permanent changes. In order to accomplish this, it is essential to know why you behave the way you do. You will also need to know why you wish to make these changes, and if you are able to adjust your life in order to accommodate them. Before simply adopting change in your life, it is essential to get to know yourself. It sounds so basic, but many people never spend the time to really know themselves.

The techniques described below are intended to help you learn more about yourself. They are only a beginning. Remember that self-awareness and self-acceptance is an ongoing, lifelong process. Traveling this road has many rewards, but there are also setbacks. Learn to enjoy the journey. For some of you, this will be relatively easy; for others, it will be extremely difficult. But I know you can do it.

When I say, "know yourself," I mean spend the time to understand your strengths and weaknesses, what motivates you, and what you like and dislike about yourself. Think about what you can and cannot change about yourself, why you behave a certain way in a certain situation, and whether deep down inside you feel that you have control over your life or that you are a victim of life's circumstances. What do you really want out of life, what are your true spiritual beliefs, what makes you happy, what makes you sad, how do you wish to be? Oprah has a great name for this. She calls it "peeling back the layers." That's what I want you to do. Take the time to explore who you are. Take as long as you like. But know yourself!

How do you begin this process? You will need a journal or a pad of paper. First, replay your life in your mind. Start as far back as you can remember. Try to recall as many major life events as you can. Pick out the three unpleasant events that you most wish you could change and write them down. See if you can answer these questions: Why were these events unpleasant? How did you react? Why did you react that way? How do you wish you had reacted? How would you react today? What has changed? What did you learn from each event? When did you learn those things?

Now recall the three most pleasant events of your life and write them down. What made these events pleasant? Where were you? Who was with you? How did you react? How would you react today? What did you learn from each event? When did you learn it?

The point of this exercise is to get you to explore your past. It may be only a beginning, but it's important to take a realistic look at your life and begin to know more about yourself. It is also important to understand that events occur in your life for a reason. It is critical that you be honest with yourself. Self-awareness means facing the facts about yourself, both good and bad. Denial is a detour that leads you nowhere. Now, let's move on to the present.

Describe yourself. Begin by writing down three things you like least about yourself. Are they things that you can change? Have you attempted to change them? How have these things affected your life? While reviewing them, accept that there are things you can change about yourself and things you cannot. But all these things serve a purpose in your life. Each one gives you an opportunity to improve yourself.

Now, write down three things you like most about yourself. Have you always had these traits? Why do you like them? How has each of these traits affected your life? Realize that each of these aspects of yourself serves a purpose in your life. Each of them also gives you the opportunity to improve yourself.

Remember that getting to know yourself is a lifetime quest.

Spend time each week or even each day discovering something about yourself. Some other questions you may want to ask yourself are:

- What makes you happy?
- What makes you sad?
- What traits do you like in others?
- What traits do you dislike in others?
- Are you a patient person?
- Are you judgmental?
- What brings you joy?
- What brings you pain?
- What are your spiritual beliefs?

Now, I want you to make a physical assessment of yourself. You can best do this in front of the mirror, with or without clothes. The purpose is not to shame you. It's to give you a true starting point from which you can work. You need to know where you are in order to know where you are going.

Picture yourself both heavier and thinner. Then say these words: "This is where I am today. I could be better. I could be worse. This represents my life."

The image you see in the mirror reflects not just your eating and exercise habits. It reflects your life. And in life, you know that nothing stays the same. Your body is no different. It's always changing. And every day, you can make a decision whether to improve it or let it slide back. This exercise should also help you understand that you have that choice.

You should try to discover something about yourself as often as possible—daily, if you can. Your journal is a great place to record the events, feelings, and emotions that occur each day.

TAKING RESPONSIBILITY

While working with people who want to lose weight, I began seeing a common philosophy among most of my clients. They usually had reasons for being overweight: an unhappy childhood, a bad marriage, an unfullfilling career, a devastating event, or a person who has caused them pain. Their reasons were always external. Something, or someone, allowed them to project the blame anywhere but on themselves.

I also noticed that the people who were successful at losing weight permanently had released all the external causes for being overweight. They accepted responsibility for it themselves. After all, you may not realize it now, and the thought may be painful at first, but you and you alone are responsible for yourself.

You create all that you are. We all have events—many of them from childhood—that have hurt us to varying degrees. But as adults we have the power to deal with those events. It is essential that you take responsibility for yourself. Take responsibility for all that you are—as well as all that you can become.

There may be people whom we blame for why we behave a certain way. I am not suggesting that some of these people were right in what they did. They need to take responsibility too. But I'm more concerned about you taking responsibility for your own life. And that means taking care of yourself. To blame people or events is a waste of time. Realize that it is usually easier to blame anything or anyone else for things that you don't like about yourself. But on the road to self-acceptance, this is a detour you cannot afford to take. Only when you assume full responsibility for yourself and your situation can you begin to accept yourself. And remember, out of self-acceptance comes self-love.

Once you understand the concept of taking responsibility for your life, it's time to move on to knowing what you really want—regarding your body, mind, and soul!

If we don't know what we want, we become like a floating balloon. Our direction in life is at the mercy of external forces. Yet it's not enough to know what we want, we have be sure we know *why* we want it. It is important to know exactly why you wish to lose weight.

The most common reason people give is that they believe it will radically change their lives. But losing weight itself will not radically change your life. I repeat, it will not! You see, what happens to most people who lose weight is that they imagine their life will suddenly be blissful and problem-free once they reach a certain weight or certain size. By the time they reach this weight, or are close to it, they realize they are still unhappy. Their unhappiness triggers their old coping mechanisms. This, in turn, leads them to put weight back on. Sadly, this is a typical weight-loss cycle.

I'll say it again: Your excess weight is a symptom of something else, maybe many things, in your life. You must come to understand what your weight represents. It may represent a void in your life or not wishing to let people down, it may represent unhappiness with yourself, it may represent unhappiness with your life. It can represent a variety of different things. But ultimately it is about not receiving enough love. And usually when this is the case, you are constantly in search of love from external sources. The secret is, it must first come from yourself.

Sandra was in search of love. She always thought it would come from marriage. But when it didn't and she realized she was unhappy in the marriage, she began to gain weight. It was only after she learned to give love to herself that the weight came off and her life changed.

Learning self-love takes time. Some people never learn it. But that is your goal. It won't happen overnight. You know you are getting closer when you take a good look at yourself one day, and despite the fact that you want to be thinner, you like yourself. To get to that point you must first know yourself. Second, you must take responsibility for yourself. Third, you must know what you want. Then you must work toward your goals.

If achieving a new body is what you want, you will find that the journey is a great way to learn self-love. That's because it is something you do for yourself. You do it because you care for yourself. And your hard work initiates a cycle of feeling physically and emotionally better.

Let's start by learning a little about how your body works. This is important for understanding and implementing the steps. Be sure you grasp these basic facts before moving on.

The Purpose of
Body Fat

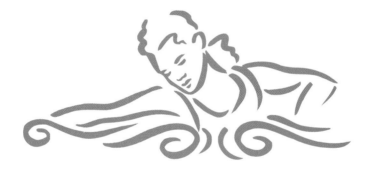

WHEN the chief of the Xhosa tribe in Africa is ready to marry, he searches for the heaviest woman in the tribe. And after they're wed, he must maintain a lifestyle that keeps his wife heavy and happy. In their culture, big is better. In American culture, the opposite is true: You can't be thin enough.

However, even here, we have had different ideas about body shape through the decades. In the 1940s and 1950s, for instance, women were exemplified by full-figured actresses such as Rita Hayworth and Jane Russell. Even into the 60s, we worshipped Marilyn Monroe—that is, until Twiggy came along. As you can see, most of the images about body type are aimed at women, but in recent years, men have been subjected to them as well. Messages about how we should look are everywhere, from film and television to advertisements. And for many of us, they leave us confused and discouraged about our bodies.

That's why it's important to shift our focus away from what others tell us about our bodies. Instead, we should be concentrating on what is most healthy for us—physically and emotionally.

The truth is, we all need to maintain a certain level of body fat to sustain life. In fact, body fat is really nothing more than stored energy. (If you have a lot of body fat, think of yourself as having a lot of energy or fuel in reserve, and our goal is to lower the amount of fuel in your tank.) Fat plays several important roles in the function of our bodies. It serves as a protective cushion for organs, provides insulation from the cold, and gives us a relatively large, efficient store of potential energy.

Not surprisingly, our bodies have a tremendous capacity to store fat. Thousands of years ago, in times of feast and famine, we hunted

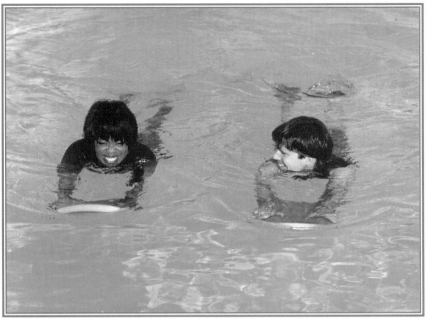

PHOTO © TIM DE FRISCO 1996

and gathered for food. The capacity to store food as fat acted as a valuable survival mechanism in times when food was scarce. But with the arrival of the agricultural revolution, when food was plentiful and we labored less for it, we began to see signs of excess weight. Now, as we move into the 21st century, obesity is at an all-time high. For most industrialized populations, food is all too abundant and calorie rich. And we hardly work to obtain it. This adds up to a lot of overweight people.

So, how much body fat do we need? A minimum of three percent of your body weight must be made up of fat for life to continue. Levels of fat this low aren't typically seen, except among highly conditioned athletes such as long-distance runners, cross-country skiers, or body-builders. For most people, I like to recommend an average percentage of body fat for women between 15 and 25 percent, and for men, between eight and 15 percent. In other words, a woman weighing 130 pounds should have between 26 and 33 pounds of body fat.

130 pounds body weight $\times$ .20 = 26 pounds body fat
130 pounds body weight $\times$ .25 = 33 pounds body fat

Your percentage of body fat can be tested by various methods such as skin fold measurements (the pinch test) or underwater weighing. With skin fold measurements, various locations on your body are pinched and measured. The measurements are then added together and a percentage of body fat, based on the total of those measurements, is obtained. Underwater weighing is considered the most accurate way to access your percentage of body fat, but I will tell you that there are relatively few labs that really know how to properly administer this test. Basically, you are placed on a hanging scale, dunked in a pool of water, and weighed while fully submerged. Your residual volume, which is a pulmonary measurement, must be measured for the test to be accurate. Skin fold measurements are routinely performed at most health clubs and by most fitness professionals. Underwater weighing is best performed at sophisticated labs, usually within universities. Some health clubs perform underwater weighing, but in general, they rarely have the proper equipment or the highly trained personnel to accurately perform this measurement.

I must tell you that many fitness professionals love to measure body fat and will usually recommend that you have this done. Unless you are a highly trained athlete or just extremely interested in these measurements, I don't recommend that you have your body fat measured. One reason is that unless performed by a highly skilled technician, these tests are fairly inaccurate. More important, when you are trying to get motivated to change your life and be comfortable with your body, the last thing you need is someone pinching your fat or dunking you in a pool of water while attached to a scale!

So how do you select your goal weight? Every year it seems, new devices or charts are on the market that tell us how much we should weigh or what our percentage of body fat should be. Every expert has his or her opinion of what you should weigh. I gave you my opinion above when I gave the body fat percentage ranges for men and women. But these ranges are approximate ranges. I believe that you should base how much weight you should lose on how you feel and how your clothes fit. If this sounds unscientific, it is! Let's face it, right now you have an idea of what your goal weight is or the ultimate size you want to be. Most people instinctively know what weight they look and feel the best at. Time and time again, when I work with a client, that client tells me the goal weight they wish to reach. This weight is almost always both within the range that I would recommend and very realistic for them to attain. I also don't recommend that you focus too much on this goal. Concentrate more on feeling good about yourself today and feeling good about the steps that you are taking toward that goal *today*. You should decide how much weight you should lose, not someone else!

Excess body fat, over and above the ideal ranges, can cause you emotional stress, leave you with a poor body image, and contribute to an increased incidence of a variety of diseases, including high blood pressure and cancer. It is well worth your time and effort to adopt a healthy lifestyle. Obviously, the answer is to modify eating habits and exercise properly. More on that later, but now let's learn how the body stores and releases fat.

The Physics of
Body Weight

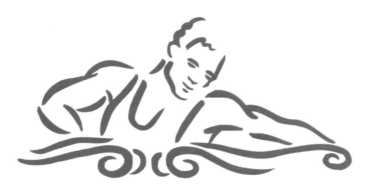

HOLD on. I know what you're thinking. You saw the word *physics* and now you're ready to skip this chapter. Don't! I'm going to keep it very simple. This information will help you understand your body and how you can change your lifestyle in order to lose weight. I think you'll find after learning these basics that the ten steps will make more sense to you.

Your body regulates everything from water and electrolytes to body temperature. Why wouldn't it regulate the storage of fat? The truth is, your body does. In fact, your body has a "set point" which controls how much fat your body maintains. Have you ever noticed how you can overeat occasionally, and, although your weight will go up, it will only increase within a certain range? Likewise, you can undereat, such as when you're on a restrictive diet. You will lose some weight, but again only to a certain extent.

Moreover, when you're on a diet, especially when it's very restrictive, you will lose only a relatively small amount of fat before your body's built-in "fat protection" mechanism kicks in. Then you start breaking down protein (muscle) and losing water weight. You see, your body can very accurately sense how many calories you are giving it. Give it a whole lot of calories and it stores some as fat, then it uses some to raise your metabolism to burn the remainder. Give your body too few calories and your metabolism shuts down, actually preventing the loss of fat while breaking down muscle. This is exactly what happened to Oprah when she did the fasting program. She lost muscle and her metabolism slowed down, making it almost impossible to maintain her weight loss. Muscle burns fat, so you certainly don't want to lose muscle. This is one reason diets don't work in the long run.

Let me explain further. The latter example shows how you lose weight—not fat—on a diet. Think of your body as being made up of two components: fat and lean mass. By lean mass, I'm referring to muscle, bone, water, and connective tissue. When you lose weight, it is possible for you to reduce fat or lean mass, or a combination of the two. Your primary goal should be to lose fat, while you maintain or increase your lean mass. Following this program will accomplish that.

And just to clear up any confusion, sometimes I use the words "weight" and "fat" synonymously. When I refer to weight loss, I actually mean the reduction of body fat. The ten steps outlined in this book are, in effect, a fat-reduction program.

As for calories, I don't think it makes a whole lot of sense to count them religiously. As I explained above, you are better off not being overly restrictive about your calories. But in the book, I will from time to time describe a particular food or snack in terms of calories to help you understand the energy values of various foods.

SET POINT

Recall that your set point regulates the amount of fat your body stores. You might ask, "Why should I change my lifestyle if my body fat is regulated by this set point?" The fact is, your set point can change. This book will show you how to decrease your set point. But first you need to learn more about it.

Your set point is determined by various genetic factors, which cannot be changed, and by your metabolism, which can be changed. Metabolism is the rate at which your body burns calories. Changing your metabolism is what this book is all about. It is the key to achieving your new body.

Think of your body as having a thermostat that can be turned up or down by modifying certain lifestyle factors. Turning up the thermo-

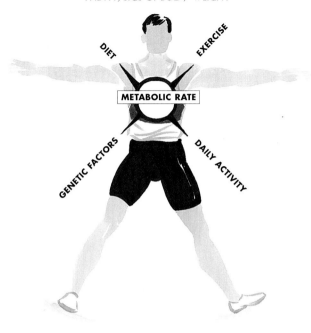

stat increases your metabolism and lowers your set point, which will allow you to release fat. Conversely, if you turn down your thermostat, you will lower your metabolism and hold on to your body fat. My goal is to give you more control over your thermostat.

Metabolism, then, has to be our focus. The concepts in this book will help you to increase your metabolism, lower your set point, and thereby decrease the amount of body fat that you store. Soon we will cover the ten steps that will accomplish this, but first you need to understand three simple concepts: the 24-hour metabolism cycle, water weight, and how and why your body weight plateaus.

THE 24-HOUR METABOLISM CYCLE

Your metabolism not only changes over the long term, it fluctuates on a daily basis. Each day your metabolism follows a predictable pattern.

Just before you wake up, your metabolism is at its slowest. It also needs to wake up! As your day proceeds, your metabolism slowly increases until it reaches its peak sometime after dinner, at which time it levels off. When you go to sleep, your metabolism gradually slows until it reaches its slowest point, which is some time just before you wake up. Then the cycle starts all over again.

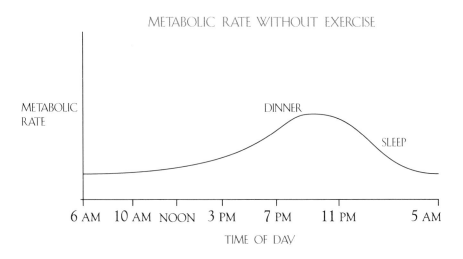

METABOLIC RATE WITHOUT EXERCISE

METABOLIC RATE

DINNER

SLEEP

6 AM   10 AM   NOON   3 PM   7 PM   11 PM   5 AM

TIME OF DAY

You can modify your 24-hour cycle to accomplish a higher over-all metabolism each day through eating and exercise. Remember that metabolism is the rate at which your body burns calories. Metabolism increases both during and after exercise, and, ironically, after eating. (Recall how I said earlier that when your body receives calories, your metabolism responds by increasing.) Therefore, if you exercise and eat soon after waking up, you will give your metabolism an earlier boost and it will remain elevated longer. This is one reason I am strongly in favor of morning exercise, as well as eating most of your calories earlier in the day.

METABOLIC RATE WITH EXERCISE

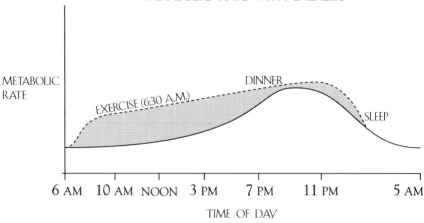

METABOLIC RATE WITH EXERCISE AND BREAKFAST

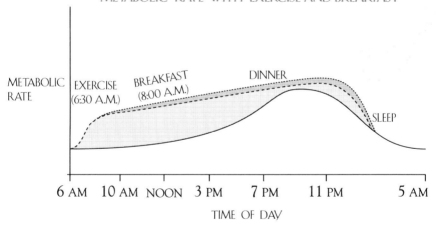

WATER WEIGHT

If you adhere to the ten steps outlined in this book, you will lose weight—primarily fat. However, there are times on a daily, weekly, and monthly basis that your body retains (and also releases) water. A considerable number of people have given up on their weight-loss regi-

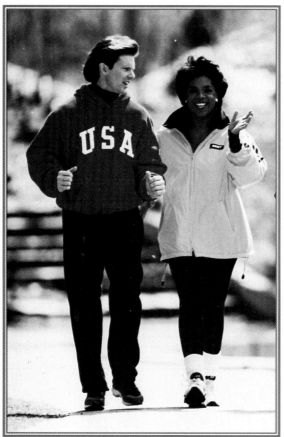

HARPO ENTERTAINMENT GROUP

men because of these nasty little jumps in water weight. The amount of these increases vary from person to person, and can account for up to seven or even eight pounds. This extra weight does not change your appearance, and should be ignored. It is only temporary. In fact, a gain in water weight often precedes a drop in your actual weight. Again, continue to follow the ten steps and ignore these minor fluctuations in your weight.

In addition to natural fluctuations in water weight, when you first start to exercise regularly or increase the amount of exercise you are already doing, your body sends out a signal to retain more water.

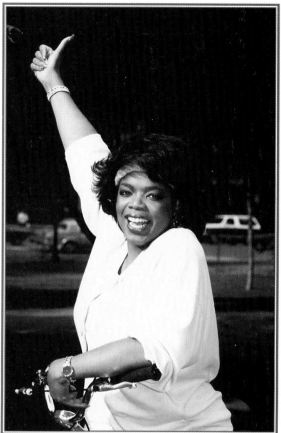

HARPO ENTERTAINMENT GROUP, PHOTO BY RICHARD SHAY

This is your body's attempt to "super hydrate" itself. Therefore, you may put on an additional two to five pounds of water weight. This can be especially bothersome in the initial weeks of your exercise program, and may fool you into thinking you have gained weight when you may have actually lost fat. Again, ignore it. Expect it to occur. But stay on your program!

I'll never forget how in the fourth week of being on the program, Oprah was ready to quit and send me on my way. Up to that point she had lost about five pounds, but when she got on the scale that week, it showed she had gained back those five and added another.

She was devastated. She had been following the plan to the letter, never cheated, and yet she put on weight. "What went wrong?" she asked me. I calmly told her not to worry, that her body was retaining fluid. Well, she didn't believe me. She even considered downing some of the diet supplement powder she had left over from another time she lost weight. But I managed to talk her out of it, and somehow she found the strength to continue with the program, even though I knew in the back of her mind she still didn't believe me. By the following week when she got on the scale, she told me I could unpack my bags. The scale showed she had not only lost the six pounds that appeared the week before, but two more.

So don't give up when the scale shows you something you don't like. It is when the results are slow or nonexistent that you will need to be the strongest.

My last point about hidden water weight is that as you become more active, you will add a small amount of muscle, which also stores its own additional water. This extra weight is "good" weight, in that it helps you to burn fat. Don't think you will become muscle-bound from the exercise—you will not. This little extra muscle weight is normal, and actually is a very good sign.

I'm reminded of another story that occurred early on in my career. I was teaching an exercise and weight-loss class that was entering its fourth week. At the end of class, one of my most dedicated participants came up to me, seemingly very frustrated. "I'm working harder than anyone in this class, and after all this time, I've gained two pounds!" she said. I knew that in addition to losing fat, she had gained a little muscle and was likely retaining a lot of water. Then, I noticed she was holding up her sweatpants. They had been tight only three weeks ago. I pointed this out to her and we both had a good laugh.

Just be sure not to fall into the trap of allowing the scale to dictate your moods. It can mislead you because of so many weight fluctuations. But it can also give you helpful information as long as you understand the concepts just discussed. I strongly recommend that you weigh yourself no more than once a week. Monday is a good day to weigh yourself because it keeps you from straying from the program during the weekend. And be consistent in how you weigh yourself. Use the same scale. Weigh yourself at the same time in the morning. And whether you weigh yourself with or without clothes, you should always do it the same way.

Once again, your body will undergo changes that you won't always understand. Do not be concerned with temporary ups or downs in your weight. Simply step back, focus on feeling better, and above all, stay on your program. Follow the ten steps and you *will* lose weight!

WHEN YOUR WEIGHT PLATEAUS

A plateau occurs when your weight remains the same for a period of time. This can last weeks or even a couple of months. With nearly every successful weight-loss program, you can expect your weight to plateau—probably many times. Plateaus occur for a variety of reasons, and are quite normal.

One of the most common reasons for a plateau is a natural adjustment to weight loss. Your body needs to make many adjustments when you lose weight, and it will release the weight only when it's ready. Realize that it is virtually impossible to lose more than three pounds of fat in a week. If you lose more than three pounds in a given week, you are losing either water weight or muscle/lean weight—which, as you know, is not what we want.

Go to the local butcher counter and ask to see three pounds of fat. You will see that it takes up a lot of space, and your body must make physical adjustments for this loss. At this time, physiologists don't know all there is to know about these adjustments, but we can be sure that they serve a purpose. Plateaus caused by these natural adjustments normally last two or three weeks, but could go on for a month or two. So be patient and stay on your program!

Another cause of plateaus is water fluctuation. As I discussed earlier, water can be retained for a variety of reasons. This extra water weight can create the illusion that you are gaining weight or have reached a plateau—even when you're losing fat. Plateaus caused by these water fluctuations typically last from three days to one week. Again, just realize that these are temporary fluctuations in your weight, and don't be alarmed.

After about six months of working with Oprah, I realized she would always lament over the extra three to four pounds she would put on at the same time each month. This was due to her menstrual cycle, so of course, she always lost the extra pounds within a few days. Finally I asked her, "Do you realize that you complain about those same four pounds, every time, every month, and you've been doing it for the last six months?" Her reply: "Oh, I guess you're right. But it still bothers me." The point is, these fluctuations may bother you too, but it's a natural occurrence. Don't let it get you sidetracked.

Cheating on your program can also cause plateaus. Let's say you've been good about following all ten steps, and you've had consistent weight loss. Now you have a bad eating and/or exercise week. This may or may not make you gain weight, but it could easily result in a prolonged plateau. This type of plateau can last as long as you are cheating on your program. My advice is to take this attitude: "Yes, I went off my program, but everyone slips up from time to time. I'm going to get right back to work and pay the price for that week."

And keep in mind, a bad day or week might not show up right away on the scale. But you shouldn't think you've gotten away with something, because it will show up at some point. This is why it's important to get right back on the program as soon as you stray from it. Don't give it up.

Finally there are "permanent" plateaus. By "permanent," I don't mean there is nothing that can be done to break through it. But given

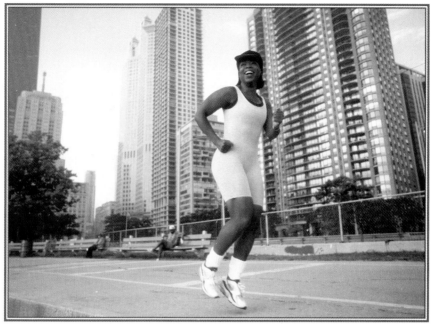

HARRY BENSON

all your current eating and exercising habits and your genetic makeup, your weight has been "re-set" at this new set point. You now have the choice of remaining at that weight, by keeping your eating and exercise program constant. Or if you desire further weight loss, you can look at each of the ten steps and start to modify one or more of them. If you understand the physics of weight loss, in particular the topics of set point and metabolism, and use and modify the steps outlined in this book, you can gain lasting control over your weight.

Now, it's time to learn the steps. You have before you a highly effective weight-loss program. Don't be intimidated. I promise that if you understand how your body works and follow the ten steps described in this book, you will have a better body and an improved self-image. Do not assume it will be easy to follow all ten steps each day for the rest of your life. It is not. But any goal worth reaching always requires hard work.

You are about to begin the first stage of the journey, which will integrate all ten steps permanently into your life. Be sure to recognize that positive changes in your life may well be connected to your new lifestyle.

Good luck, and let's get started!

The Ten Steps

*H*aving tried a gajillion diets, I understand how when we want to lose weight, we tend to look for the answer outside ourselves. We want a magic solution—a secret formula. I used to wish somebody would just tell me the answer—show me the way. Someone did. But I've also learned what Glenda, the good witch, told Dorothy in The Wizard of Oz, "You always had it. You always had the power." The real secret is within you. These ten steps can show you the way. They can bring you home to yourself.

—**Oprah**

1. Exercise aerobically, five to seven days each week (preferably in the morning).

2. Exercise in the zone (at a level seven or eight).

3. Exercise for 20 to 60 minutes each exercise session.

4. Eat a low-fat, balanced diet each day.

5. Eat three meals and two snacks each day.

6. Limit or eliminate alcohol.

7. Stop eating two to three hours before bedtime.

8. Drink six to eight glasses of water each day.

9. Have at least two servings of fruit and three servings of vegetables each day.

10. Renew your commitment to healthy living each day (Daily Renewal).

THESE are the ten most effective and most efficient changes you can make to increase your metabolism and lose weight. Adopt them into your life, and you will have a healthier body and mind.

The tough part is finding the discipline, inner strength, and willpower to carry out the ten steps. There are plenty of shortcuts out there. Some even work—temporarily. But following the ten steps daily is the way to permanent weight loss.

Most of the steps are basic principles. You may even be using some of them in your life already. That's good. But it's the combination of these ten steps that makes them a powerful and permanent program for weight loss.

You may be wondering, why these ten. It's a question I'm often asked. I developed these ten steps over the past fifteen years through a combination of studying how metabolism works and my experience in working with a variety of people to achieve their fitness and weight-loss goals. Part of my philosophy is theoretical, since metabolism itself is very difficult to study. As you learned previously, metabolism is the rate at which your body uses calories. Metabolism cannot be directly measured in a lab. It is only estimated, and not with a great degree of accuracy. But realize that a small change in your metabolism will result in a large change in your percentage of body fat.

The most valuable contribution to the development of this program came from my work with people. One of my first clients was a man named George. I was so inspired by him. You see, George was a heart transplant patient. At the time, I was astounded that someone could receive the heart of another person and lead such a productive life. Not only was his life productive, but he continually showed a desire and commitment to improve upon it. In rehabilitation class, he was always positive and helped other patients. He followed his workout program to the letter, but he also worked just a little bit harder than everyone else. And on days I knew he didn't feel his best, he never once acted bitter about his situation. There was a certain peace about George. He progressed at twice the pace of anyone in the class, yet his starting condition was much more serious than most. I was sorry to see him leave after he finished his therapy. As he walked out the door, I asked him what he was doing for Easter break, and he said, "I'm hiking the Canyon." He meant the Grand Canyon. I learned from George that it is possible to achieve just about anything if you want to.

For several years, I continued to work with heart patients who needed to lose weight to improve their health. I kept noticing that the ones who worked just a little bit harder lost weight faster and had a higher rate of success overall. They got fit, began eating healthier, and stuck to the program I had outlined for them. The ones who didn't work quite as hard saw fewer results, became disheartened, and sometimes dropped their program. It seemed there was a "zone" that existed. And when clients exercised consistently within this zone, results soon followed.

When coupled with the science behind metabolism, this zone makes sense. Look at a simple cell. When you exercise at a high rate, the cell responds by using oxygen at a faster rate. That means it's burning more calories. If you train your cells to work at this faster rate by exercising intensely on a daily or almost daily basis, then they will always burn calories at a higher rate. You will change your metabolism. Now you can see how steps one and two evolved. The rest of the steps evolved in much the same way, using real-life experiences backed by scientific theory.

The other question I'm often asked is why I chose to specialize in working with people who drastically want or need to change their lives. I didn't always know the answer to that. Now I do. Midway through my career I began working solely with weight-loss patients.

Most people in my field long to work with athletes. But I was always more interested in the people who seemed to most need my help. A lot of these people were depressed and filled with desperation. I was familiar with their struggles. Many of my family members battle with their weight.

I can remember being eight years old and going to visit my great-grandmother. She never once greeted me at the door. Instead I would go to her bedroom, which was once the dining room, and climb up on her bed and kiss her on the cheek. My great-grandmother was too large to leave her bed. I once asked my mother why "Mom-Mom" was always in bed. She told me that my great-grandmother had hurt her knee many years ago. Of course, it wasn't until I began working with people who needed to lose a lot of weight that I realized it was about more than just her knee. Surprisingly, she lived to be 92. I think of her often. I'm sure she influenced my choice of careers.

Now, I can't imagine doing anything else for a living. I want to share my experience and this program with you. You are about to incorporate ten powerful steps into your life.

Steps one through nine directly or indirectly affect your metabolism. Step ten is motivational. When performed together, these ten steps have always resulted in dramatic weight loss. Think of the steps as an insurance policy for the future—you need to pay just a small premium each day to ensure a healthy body for life. The steps interact with each other to further boost your metabolism and, consequently, your weight-loss results. I also chose them because they can be done each day, without drastically altering your life. And there is little or no cost in carrying out each of these steps. In short, these are ten of the best things you can do for your health—and your life.

This is not to say that there aren't other activities you can adopt to help you lose weight. For example, I know that weight training or weight lifting is a valuable activity to promote and maintain weight loss, especially in the long run. It has other health benefits as well, such as prevention of osteoporosis. I think weight training is extremely worthwhile. I usually introduce it to my weight-loss clients about three months after they start the program, and only then when I'm certain they have firmly incorporated the ten steps into their lives.

There will be some of you who are able to achieve weight loss by adopting fewer than all ten steps. However, you should picture each of the ten steps as links in a chain—the chain is only as strong as the weakest link. I strongly recommend that you use all ten, since this will not only give you the most effective weight-loss program, but will also significantly improve your overall health. Some of the steps have been shown to decrease the risk of various cancers, lessen the chances of a heart attack, lower blood pressure, and reduce psychological stress.

Within the guidelines of most of the steps, there is a minimum and maximum level of performance. My recommendation is that you start out with the minimum. Once you've implemented all ten steps, wait to see what your weight does. Be sure to give yourself enough time for results to occur. If you feel you have reached a permanent plateau, which we talked about previously, consider raising your level of performance within the steps. For example, step three is exercise for 20 to 60 minutes each exercise session. The minimum requirement for this step is 20 minutes. So start there and add minutes after all the other nine steps are met daily and when you feel you're ready to exercise longer. As for the maximum of 60 minutes, there really should not be a reason to exercise over 60 minutes unless you are training for an endurance event.

Also, the ten steps should be used on a daily basis. When performed daily, the net result is always weight loss. I don't claim that these steps will be easy to adopt permanently. They won't. The key to performing them is finding the discipline to carry them out each day and recognizing the many ways they benefit your life. If you perform these ten steps consistently, you will lose weight—and more important, you will gain control over your weight. You will change your life.

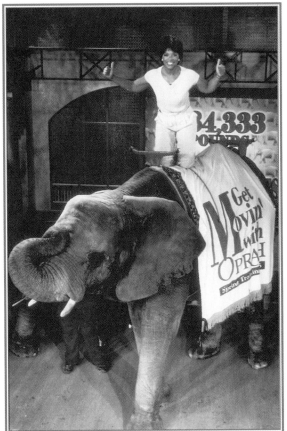

HARPO ENTERTAINMENT GROUP

A WORD BEFORE YOU BEGIN

The phrase "consult your physician prior to beginning an exercise program" seems to appear on virtually every exercise video, exercise program, exercise book, and piece of exercise equipment available. We see this or a similar phrase so often that I believe we completely ignore the message and assume that it is a statement regarding liability.

Certainly, it does serve this function, but it's also great advice! Checking with your physician can uncover medical conditions that need attention before you start your exercise program. These include high cholesterol and high blood pressure (which should be brought under control) and smoking (which should be given up). And if you are immediately "cleared," you'll have the peace of mind of knowing you can safely exercise at recommended levels.

Your physician can also help select activities that are appropriate, given your specific health concerns. Finally, consulting your physician establishes a level of communication that is helpful for you and your doctor in assessing your entire health and medical profile.

So check with your physician soon, and get ready to move!

Step One

EXERCISE AEROBICALLY, FIVE TO SEVEN DAYS EACH WEEK

(PREFERABLY IN THE MORNING)

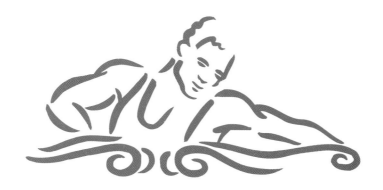

*had given up on exercise. I would sporadically try it at the begin-
ning of every year—you know, New Year's resolution. I remember
running at the beginning of January 1993—two months before I
started working with Bob. I was with a friend and I told her, "I really don't
believe in exercise." "Then why are you doing it?" she replied. "Only
because they say it's supposed to work, but I think they're all lying." You
see, I had been doing it off and on for years and it hadn't done one thing
for me but make me tired. I'd see women working out, wearing those cute
little thongs and I'd think, must be nice to have good genes and such a good
metabolism. I now know that many of those same woman were blessed
with good genes, but many of them worked hard to achieve a formidable
metabolism.*

*It was exciting news to me to know that with regular exercise (not
the three days a week we always heard about, I mean 5–7 days a week) I
could change my metabolism. And a good metabolism is what you need to
burn fat.*

*For years I'd dieted and occasionally got moving, but I wasn't moving
enough. I was never consistent. Now I work out seven days a week—it's
as natural as brushing my teeth. A lot of days I don't enjoy doing it. I'm
not one of those people who can claim they love to exercise. But I do love
all it does for me.*

—Oprah

I had just arrived in Chicago to begin working with Oprah. It was
about five P.M., Oprah had already taped two shows and attended a
number of meetings, and we were just completing our first workout.

She was still sweating and catching her breath, but now was the time to tell her what she would need to do to reach her goal weight and stay there. "You will have to exercise six or seven days a week," I said. "And you'll need to do it in the morning." I was already preparing myself for her objections.

Without hesitating, Oprah looked me in the eye and said, "Okay, I'll see you at five-fifteen in the morning." I was ecstatic. I knew then that she would be successful and lose the weight.

Unfortunately, Oprah's reaction is unusual. Just think of what your reaction was when you first read step one. Of all ten steps, this is the one that usually meets the most resistance. Yet, it is one of the most important steps.

When I worked with Oprah on a series of shows on fitness in spring 1995, I observed that the most successful participants were people who viewed exercise as "part of their day." And that's what I want you to do. You probably know that exercise is essential for long-term weight-loss success. What I want to instill in you is that exercise needs to take place daily, or close to it, for it to have a long-lasting effect on your metabolism. This makes more sense if you remember the 24-hour metabolism cycle. You want to heat up the body on a daily basis to permanently affect your metabolism. You also want to increase the amount of aerobic enzymes in your muscles—these little buggers will help you burn fat more effectively 24 hours a day.

I can understand why some of you might be confused about how often you should exercise. You have probably heard that you need to exercise a minimum of three times a week for results. My question is, for what type of results? Three times a week will improve your health and your cardiovascular system, and you'll even feel much better. But it doesn't do enough to change your metabolism and vastly reduce your weight. This is the reason you need to get aerobic exercise daily, or at least five times a week, to have dramatic and lasting weight-loss results. In fact, I won't take on weight-loss clients unless they are willing to exercise aerobically a minimum of five times a week. Are you willing?

EXERCISE IN THE MORNING

There are several reasons why I want you to exercise first thing in the morning. The initial reason is purely physiological. When you exercise in the morning, you are charging up your metabolism right from the start. This keeps your metabolism elevated throughout the day, so that you burn extra calories even when you're not exercising. Just think about all those calories you'll burn while sitting at your desk. If you wait until the afternoon or early evening to exercise, your metabolism tapers off much sooner, and you lose the benefit of burning extra calories.

The second reason is entirely psychological. Morning exercise does not allow for excuses—and you know we are all masters at finding excuses not to exercise. There are a million reasons that can come up in the course of a day: The kids need to be picked up, you have an important meeting, you're running late, the dog got sick. You get the picture. These excuses are part of the reason exercise professionals have observed that only 25 percent of all evening exercisers are consistent with their programs, as opposed to 75 percent of morning exercisers.

Exercise is also a more effective stress reducer when you do it in the morning. When you begin to exercise in the morning, you will notice that you are better able to handle stress and crises throughout your day.

Finally, morning exercise will help you focus on your new lifestyle. By putting it first in your day, it will act as a daily reminder that this way of life is a priority to you, which, in turn, will help you to

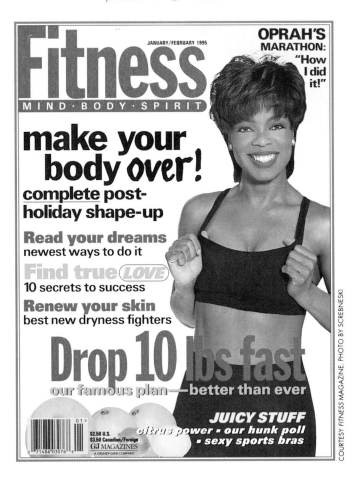

stay on track with your eating steps for the rest of the day. Morning exercise is also more conducive to renewing yourself. We'll talk more about daily renewal in step ten.

For all of the previously mentioned reasons, when I work with a new client who is used to exercising in the evening, I go to great lengths to convert them to morning exercise. You remember Louise,

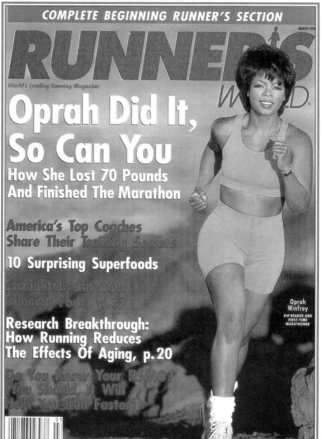

the stock trader. She was exercising in the evenings because she felt that was most convenient. When I met her, I explained that she would benefit more by working out in the morning, because not only would it boost her metabolism but it would help reduce some of the stress she faced on her job. Louise explained to me that in order to exercise in the morning, she would have to wake up at 4:30 A.M. So I countered with, "How bad do you want to lose those twelve pounds?" Now she loves working out in the morning.

So prepare to wake up and get moving!

AEROBIC VS. ANAEROBIC

You've probably heard the term "aerobic" exercise, and maybe you're wondering what it really means. Aerobic simply means "with oxygen." Exercises that require a lot of oxygen are called "aerobic." They are different from exercises that are "anaerobic," which means "in the absence of oxygen." (The primary energy source required for this exercise is stored in muscle and comes from a process called glycolosis—if you're interested!)

Many people assume that an exercise is either entirely aerobic (such as running or cross-country skiing) or entirely anaerobic (throwing a shot put or weight training). That's really not the case. Virtually every exercise uses energy from your aerobic system as well as your anaerobic system. But different exercises use different amounts of oxygen. Our goal is to select exercises that are primarily aerobic.

When you perform a highly aerobic exercise on a regular basis, such as walking or jogging, you are increasing your aerobic enzymes. Aerobic enzymes will help you burn more fat, so you want a lot of them. In general, the more aerobic an exercise is, the greater effect it will have on your aerobic enzymes and your metabolism and, ultimately, your weight.

Now, let me say a few things about weight training. I'm sure some of you have been told that it is beneficial to lift weights while you're trying to lose pounds. It is beneficial. But all too often, by lifting weights you are less willing to devote the necessary time to your aerobic exercise. After all, you only have so much time and energy.

This makes me think of a woman I know at a health club I often visit. When I first saw her working out with her trainer two years ago, she would spend ten minutes on the treadmill followed by an hour of lifting weights. She weighed about 350 pounds. I assumed when she was on the treadmill, she was cooling down from the aerobic portion of her workout session. It wasn't until recently that I realized the ten minutes on the treadmill was her aerobic workout. Today, this woman is still at least 350 pounds. I'm amazed that she is still willing to show up at the gym after not having lost one pound in two years. I really feel badly for her. What this woman needs to do is focus on raising her metabolism and increasing her aerobic enzymes. And to do that, she needs to perform aerobic exercises. She can add weight training later.

Weight training (lifting) is primarily an anaerobic exercise. To make it more aerobic, the concept of circuit weight training became popular a number of years ago. Circuit weight training involves moving quickly from weight machine to weight machine, usually performing the exercises more rapidly. Although this type of weight training may be slightly more aerobic than traditional weight training, you are fooled into thinking you are exercising more aerobically than you really are. That's because weight training elevates your heart rate, but it does not use a lot of oxygen compared to say, jogging, and, consequently, does not increase your aerobic enzymes. In the short run, you are doing little to change your metabolism. That's why I do not consider circuit weight training an aerobic exercise. It should not be used to satisfy this step.

Weight training does, however, have other benefits, mainly increasing and retaining muscle mass, strengthening joints and ligaments, and maintaining bone density. It can also improve your metabolism in the long run—by building and retaining muscle. You should seriously consider it as an adjunct activity once you have incorporated all of the other steps into your life and feel you have adequate time to devote to it.

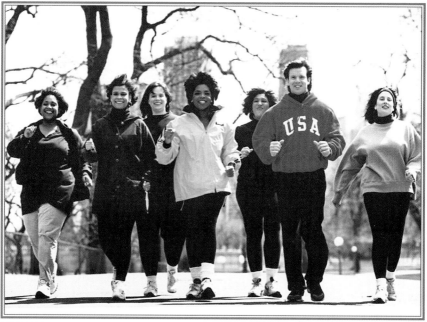

HARPO ENTERTAINMENT GROUP

CHOOSING A PRIMARY EXERCISE

Since you will be exercising at least five times a week, you will need to select a form of aerobic exercise that you can live with and, yes, maybe even enjoy. In setting up your typical week of exercise, I strongly recommend that you choose a primary exercise, as well as one or two alternate exercises.

Your primary exercise should be one you can readily do—even when you're away from home. It will become the exercise you are most highly trained in. You will do this exercise at least three to four times a week. (Remember, I am asking you to exercise at least five times each week.) Your alternate exercise(s) will make up the difference. Your alternate can help you tone different muscles and keep you from getting bored.

Your primary exercise must be highly aerobic, relatively easy to perform, and convenient. For example, cross-country skiing is highly aerobic, but it's not easy to learn for most people. And outdoor cross-country skiing is not at all convenient, since you need to live where there is constant snow on the ground. Based on these and other considerations, I have found four exercises that qualify as primary exercises:

Walking
Jogging
Aerobic Dance
Stair stepping

Walking

Walking is my top choice for most of you who want to lose weight. It is highly aerobic; you don't have to learn a new skill; you don't need any expensive equipment; and you can perform it just about anywhere. In addition, walking does not place a lot of stress on your muscles and joints. It's one of the only highly aerobic exercises that you can perform each day of the week without great risk of overuse injuries. You are also not required to select alternate activities, although it's still a good idea to add some variety to your week. For all of these reasons, the majority of my clients start out walking. Some progress to jogging or aerobic dance; others stick with walking. It will be up to you.

A recent client of mine weighed 211 pounds when she started this program. There was no question in my mind that the best exercise for her was walking, and that she would always need to use walking as her primary exercise because of an old knee injury. Just by walking she has already dropped more than 50 pounds. She has another ten to go to reach her goal. And, for her, walking works just fine.

If you choose walking as your primary exercise, you want to be

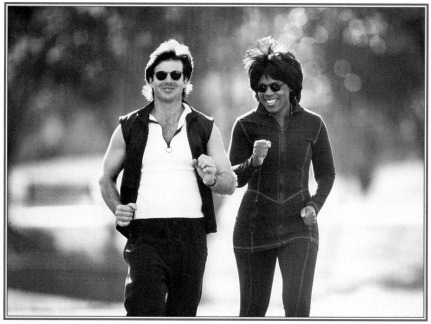

© TIM DE FRISCO 1996

sure you are aerobically walking and not just strolling. There is a distinct difference between the two. To properly perform the technique of aerobic walking, good posture is essential. It is important to keep your head straight and chin up and to look forward, not down. Keep your shoulders up and level—not hunched or rolled forward. Your hips should be in line with your shoulders, and your back should be erect. Bend your arms at a 90-degree angle and swing them to help propel you as you walk. As you swing your arms, make sure that your hands don't reach above shoulder level. Refer to the illustration for proper and improper form. And remember, the more you walk, the better your form will become!

Use the checklist below to help you with the technique for aerobic walking:

1. Use good posture

2. Head up, chin straight

3. Shoulders out and aligned with hips

4. Chest out

5. 90-degree arm swing

6. Breathing is performed primarily through your mouth, not your nose

The pace or intensity that you walk at is determined by your level of fitness. This is covered in detail in Step Two. Oprah started out walking at a pace of 17 minutes per mile. She quickly progressed to 13 minutes per mile. If you select walking as your primary exercise, you will notice that you become faster as time goes by. This is a sign that good things

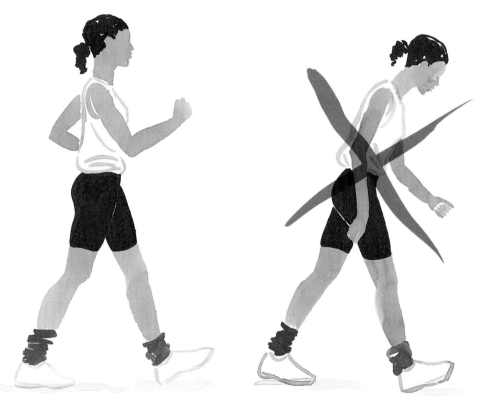

are happening. You are working harder and you are losing weight. I have seen individuals go from a starting pace of over 26 minutes per mile to under 12 minutes per mile. And always, their weight dropped as their minutes per mile fell. Start out concentrating on good form, then focus on walking at a level that will bring you results.

Jogging

Once Oprah was walking at a 13-minute-mile pace, she then switched to jogging as her primary exercise, and walking became one of her alternates. Because of Oprah's set point (remember, this regulates the amount of fat your body stores), she needed to progress to jogging to continue losing weight. Many of you will be able to reach your goal weight by remaining with walking as your primary exercise.

But if you decide to make jogging your primary activity, there are a few things you should know. On the positive side, jogging typically produces the fastest weight-loss results, is easy to learn, can be performed just about anywhere, and doesn't require a great deal of expense.

On the other hand, jogging places a lot of stress on your body—muscles, ligaments, and joints in particular. If you're prone to orthopedic problems, such as strains or sprains of the knee, ankle, or hip, jogging may not be for you. In addition, jogging places more stress on your cardiovascular system, which may create a problem for people with high blood pressure or other heart and pulmonary complications. Asthma may present another concern. And, if you need to lose a considerable amount of weight, jogging places even more stress on your body, and walking is probably a better choice. Your physician or a qualified exercise specialist can help you decide.

The primary difference between walking and jogging is that in walking, one foot is always in contact with the ground. In jogging, you push off the ground with your back leg, so that you are actually airborne for a split second.

Jogging also emphasizes different muscles than walking does. Actually, the two can complement each other well. By using a technique that combines walking and jogging, you can get the benefits of both. You simply walk for a while, then jog. When you become tired, return to walking. This is a good technique to use if your weight has reached a permanent plateau with walking alone, and you don't want to jump right into jogging for your entire workout.

Like walking, there is a proper way to jog. For most of us, jogging is a natural activity to perform, and, with consistent participation, we usually adopt good form. Refer to the illustrations below for proper jogging form and on page 110 for improper jogging form.

1. Use good posture—head up, look straight ahead

2. Keep shoulders square, slightly ahead of hips

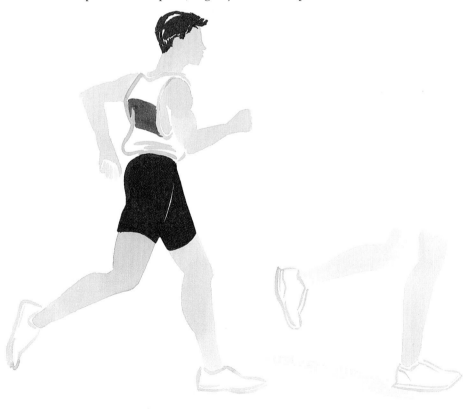

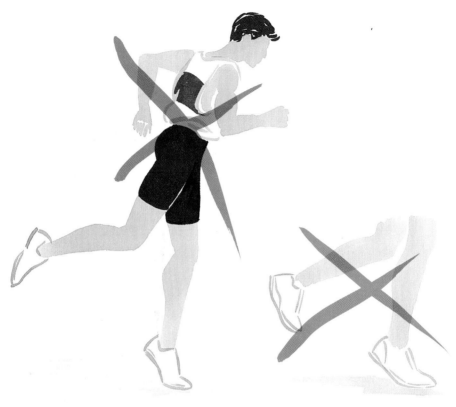

3. Swing arms freely at about a 90-degree angle

4. Let hands hang loosely, move freely

5. Strike the ground with heel of your foot

6. Breathing is performed primarily through your mouth, not your nose

Because of the stress to your body, you should only jog a maximum of four times a week. You will need to fulfill step one by making up the difference with your alternate exercise.

And, again, as is the case with walking, you should increase your pace according to your ability. Keep in mind, as you become faster your weight will drop.

Aerobic Dance

Aerobic dance, or aerobics, provides what its name implies, a highly aerobic activity. The traditional aerobics class format uses basic dance steps to improve cardiovascular fitness, as well as to tone up muscles. Now there are many different variations, such as step aerobics, cardio-funk, jazzercise, slide aerobics, water aerobics, even boxing aerobics. As you can see, aerobics classes can offer a fun way to exercise. If properly taught, most aerobics classes can also offer a good workout option. Even your warm-up, stretching, and cool down are built into the class. (I'll say more about those later.) But some classes are better than others. For example, water aerobics can be taught as an aerobic activity, but the water prevents your body from heating up as it would in other aerobics classes. That's why I don't recommend water aerobics as a primary exercise.

If you choose aerobic dance as your primary exercise, there are some other things you should consider. Soon after the aerobics craze hit, instructors began seeing a lot of overuse injuries in muscles and joints. Then they were able to lower the impact of the exercise without sacrificing much of the aerobic benefits. Today, most classes are low in impact, even if they are high in intensity. Still, I believe some injuries can occur if you are taking aerobics classes more than four times a week. I recommend you do them only three times a week, four at the most, and choose at least one alternate exercise to complete Step One.

Also consider what it will cost you to pay for classes or join a facility that offers them. Obviously you want to find a class you enjoy and one that is convenient. Once you find an instructor you like, keep in mind that the quality of your workout will depend on that instructor remaining at your facility and your attending classes. If you are often away from home, this might not be a good choice for you.

The best recommendation I can make if you use aerobic dance as your primary exercise is to find a class you like and one that is taught by a qualified, motivating instructor. I recommend that the instructor be certified by ACE (American Council on Exercise) or AFAA (Aerobics and Fitness Association of America).

Stair Stepping

Stair stepping is another activity you can choose as your primary exercise. Though you can do this on a step machine or by climbing a staircase or by using steps at a stadium, I will mainly focus on the proper way of using a machine, since that is the most common way this exercise is done today.

Stair stepping has several pluses. First, it puts little stress on your body. In addition, it is relatively easy to learn. Finally, since it is primarily an indoor activity, it is not dependent on the weather.

But stair stepping is not as aerobic as the first three activities listed. That's because when you step on a machine, you are not moving all of your body weight—the stepper supports some of it. You are also using fewer muscles than any of the other three primary exercises.

Stair stepping also requires you to either buy a relatively expensive piece of equipment (the inexpensive steppers are a waste of time!) or to join a health club that has step machines.

I have seen a lot of people use step machines incorrectly. By using the proper form, you can maximize the aerobic benefit of this exercise. Refer to the illustrations on pages 113 and 114.

Use the checklist below to help you with your stepping technique:

1. Use good posture

2. Head up, chin straight

3. Shoulders back

4. Hands in contact with machine

5. Arms should be bent and not supporting your weight

6. Take medium to large steps

And keep in mind that your hands should be in contact with the stepper for balance, not to support your weight.

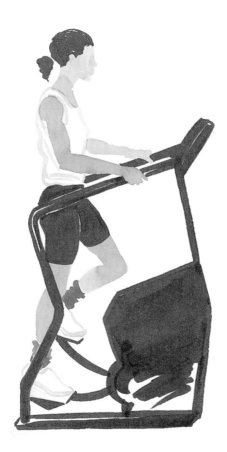

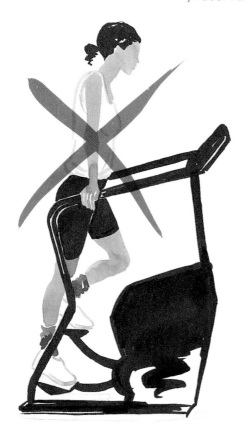

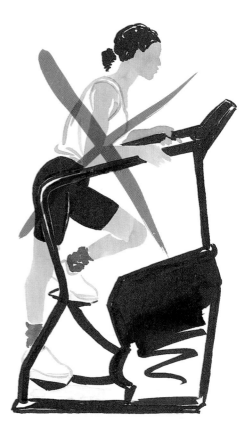

CHOOSING ALTERNATE ACTIVITIES

If you selected any activity other than walking for your primary activity, you will need to choose at least one alternate activity. Even if walking is your primary activity, it is a good idea to add a little variety into your program.

The best choice for your alternate activity would be one of the four exercises just covered—walking, jogging, aerobic dance, or stair stepping. But for more diversity, I have listed some others. I chose them based on their aerobic potential, ease of learning and performing, and convenience. I am not saying these are the only activities you should use, but I think they are the best. They are:

Outdoor cycling
Stationary cycling
Rowing
Cross-country skiing
Swimming

Outdoor Cycling

Outdoor cycling is a moderately aerobic activity. But mostly, it's downright fun! That's the main reason I recommend it. You can also use it to get to a destination, and you can enjoy it with other people.

There are a few things to keep in mind, though. First, cycling has a high injury rate from accidents. So it's important to find a route that has minimal traffic. You should choose a course without a lot of stop signs or stop lights.

You might also have to buy a bike, and these days a good quality one is fairly expensive. Another thing to keep in mind is that the bike supports most of your weight, making cycling less aerobic than the four primary activities.

If you cycle, I recommend that you double the time of your pri-

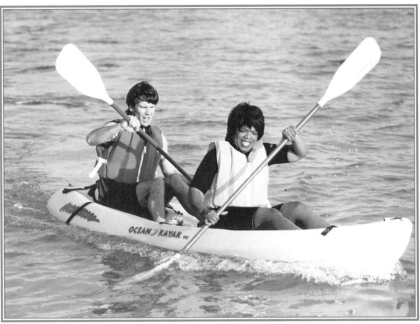

© TIM DE FRISCO 1996

mary exercise. In other words, if you usually stair step for 20 minutes, you will need to cycle for 40 minutes to get the same result. If you have been walking for 60 minutes, that means you need to cycle for two hours. You get the idea.

Finally, with cycling, you are at the mercy of the weather. And don't forget to wear your helmet!

Stationary Cycling

Stationary cycling is aerobic enough to be considered an alternate activity—though just barely. This activity is slightly less aerobic than outdoor cycling because there is no wind resistance. Nor are you propelling your weight forward as you do in outdoor cycling. You can partly overcome this by changing the resistance on your stationary cycle.

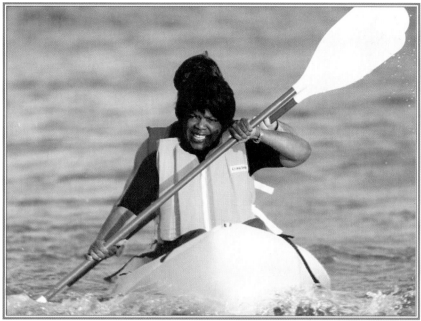

© TIM DE FRISCO 1996

Among the negatives for this exercise, you will again need to double your exercise time, you might have to buy a stationary bicycle (though there is a device that converts a regular bike), and you may become bored by the repetitive motion and lack of scenery. On the positive side, stationary cycling is easy to perform, you don't have to worry about the weather, it does not place a lot of stress or pounding on your body, and you can do other things while cycling, such as read or watch television (although don't forget to maintain your proper intensity, which is covered in step two).

Rowing

Rowing, whether performed inside on a stationary rower, or outdoors in a specialized rowing boat, provides you with an excellent aerobic activity. It places little stress on the joints and ligaments, can be performed indoors or out, and conditions both your upper and lower body. Some boats are better than others, however. A rowing shell is best for an all-over body workout, whereas in a kayak your arms do most of the work. As for canoes, you are barely using your legs at all. Save it for recreation, after your workout.

If you take up this activity, you may have to buy some equipment and spend some time learning how to properly use it. And you should know, some people find indoor rowing a bit boring.

Cross-Country Skiing

Here's another exercise that can be performed indoors or out. Cross-country skiing is a highly aerobic activity that trains both your arms and legs. There is also little stress placed on the muscles, joints, and ligaments. And it is relatively safe—especially on an indoor ski machine.

The disadvantages to cross-country skiing include the cost to outfit yourself. It also helps to be moderately fit to fully benefit from this activity. And you must learn and practice an intricate skill that requires coordination and balance.

Working out on an indoor ski machine is not as aerobic as skiing outdoors. And you might find it a little boring. On the other hand, if you're skiing outdoors, you'll need enough snow on the ground.

Swimming

I consider swimming a moderately aerobic activity. Overall, it's one of the least stressful exercises for your body. It can be pleasant, fun, and refreshing. Personally, I love it. But swimming barely passes as an alternate activity.

There are a number of drawbacks to swimming. The water's cool temperature prevents your body from heating up as much as it would in other activities. And this will limit the impact on your metabolism.

It may also affect your appetite. Most triathletes will tell you that on days when they are cycling or running, they won't feel hungry for a few hours. But on swim days, they are ready to eat almost as soon as they leave the pool. Though it hasn't been fully documented, some exercise physiologists, including myself, think that an elevated body temperature depresses your appetite. Swimming does not significantly elevate your body temperature. Just think of when you have a fever; you usually don't feel much like eating. It's the same principle.

The other drawback to swimming has to do with body fat. The more fat you carry on your body, the more you float and the less you work.

For all these drawbacks, I think you should only occasionally use swimming as an alternate exercise. It is, however, an excellent activity to use while you are recovering from an orthopedic injury.

A WORD ABOUT RECREATIONAL SPORTS

You might be wondering about sports, such as racquetball, tennis, handball, and basketball. These are for recreation. They should not be used for a workout session. Each sport has active phases and resting phases. The resting phases break the continuous flow of aerobic activity.

Your workouts will allow you to participate in these sports at a higher level. So enjoy them, but also be sure to get in your workout!

STRETCHING

Stretching is the forgotten child of fitness. It is the one area Oprah goes to great lengths to skip. She can be quite creative with her rea-

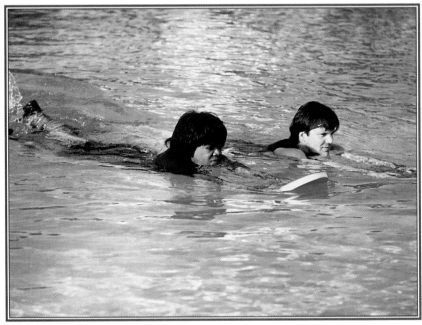

© TIM DE FRISCO 1996

sons. I wish I had an accurate number of how many exercisers actually stretch. I would guess under 30 percent.

Nevertheless, I am hoping to convince you to stretch. Evidence suggests that stretching can reduce the risk of injury to muscles, ligaments, and joints, as well as improve your athletic performance. It also helps to relax and mentally prepare you for your exercise session. And once you build it into your routine, it really feels good!

The technique of stretching has evolved over the years. A couple of decades ago, stretching was performed ballistically (bouncing up and down). This was found to create as many problems as it solved. A static method then became popular. You hold your stretch for anywhere between 15 seconds to two minutes. This technique is still the standard method for stretching and is quite effective.

But I prefer a technique that takes the static method even further. It involves holding each stretch for one to four seconds, relaxing

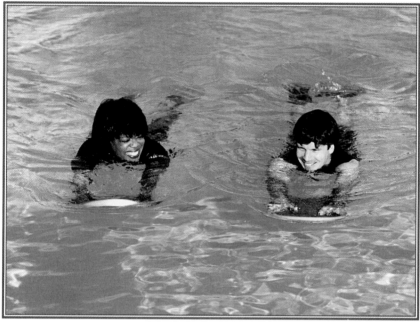

© TIM DE FRISCO 1996

for two to six seconds and again stretching for one to four seconds. This pattern is repeated for about two minutes for each stretch. I consider this the method of choice.

Each fitness expert has a slightly different approach to stretching, but the point remains the same: *Stretch before you exercise!*

My personal approach:

Always warm up *before* you stretch. To do so, walk or march until you are slightly warm. Then perform a stretch for each major muscle group using alternating stretching and relaxing phases. Refer to the illustrations on the following pages.

Hold each stretch for one to four seconds, relax for two to six seconds, stretch and hold again for one to four seconds. Perform each stretch for about two minutes. Stretch for five to ten minutes before your exercise session and for five to ten minutes after your session. Don't bounce. Breathe comfortably while you stretch.

Recommended stretches include:

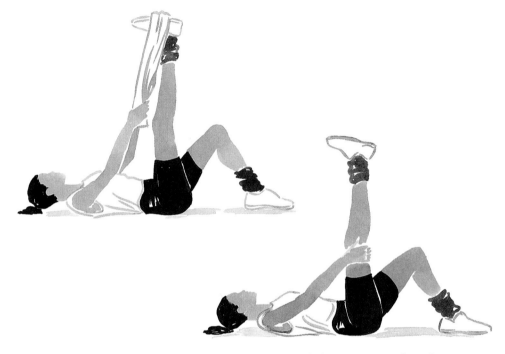

Lie on your back, keeping one leg bent and the corresponding foot on the floor. Raise your other leg up, assisting with your hands or using a towel to assist, until you feel a gentle tension in the hamstring. Repeat on the other side.

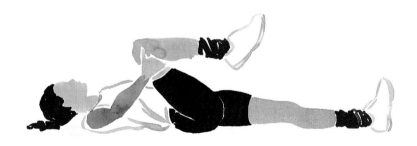

While lying on your back, grab the back of your leg just above the knee, gently pull that leg up toward your chest. Keep your opposite leg straight on the ground. Repeat on the other side.

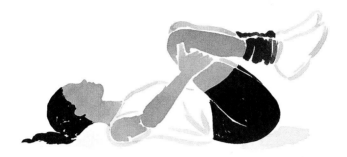

While lying on your back, grab the back of both legs just above the knee, and pull them up toward your chest.

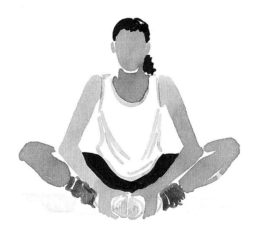

While sitting on the floor, place the soles of your feet together and allow your knees to drop down toward the floor. Gradually pull your feet toward you, until you feel gentle tension in your inner thighs and groin. You can lean forward as you become more flexible.

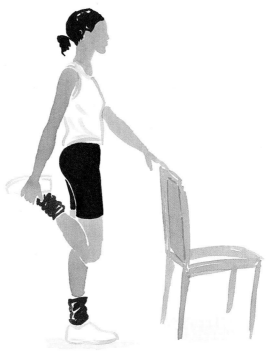

While holding on to something for support, grab your ankle and bend your leg behind you, bringing your heel up toward your buttocks until you feel gentle tension in the front of your thigh. The closer you can bring your heel to your buttocks, the more flexible you are. Be sure to bend slightly on the opposite leg and keep your knees aligned. Repeat for the other leg.

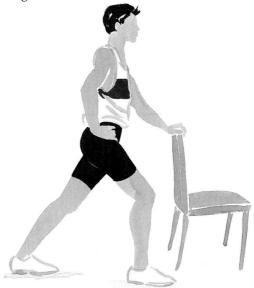

While holding on to something for support with one hand, place the other hand on your hip. Extend one leg straight out behind you, with your heel on the ground. The opposite leg is bent in front of you while keeping the knee directly over the corresponding foot (not ahead of it). The stretch should be felt in the upper calf of the leg that is straight back. If you don't feel it, bring the leg in front (the one that's bent) further forward. Again, you should feel gentle tension. Be sure not to arch your back. Repeat on the other side.

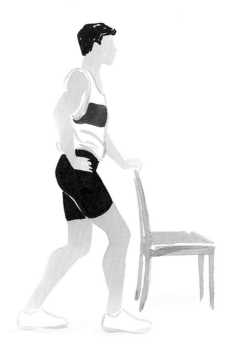

While holding on to something for support with one hand, place the other hand on your hip. One foot is slightly ahead of the other and your knees are bent. Bring your hips slowly down toward the floor, keeping both heels on the ground. You should feel gentle tension in the lower calf of the leg that is back. Do not arch your back. Repeat on the other side.

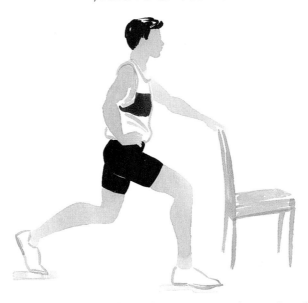

While holding on to something for support with one hand, place the other hand on your hip, keeping your head, neck, shoulders, back, and hips aligned. With one leg in front and the other behind, gradually drop in a straight line down toward the floor. Your front knee should be kept in line with your front ankle—not ahead of it. Gentle tension should be felt in the hip of the back leg. You can accentuate the stretch by slightly rolling your hips forward. Repeat on the other side.

For an upper-body stretch, stand with your head, shoulders, and hips aligned and your hands clasped behind you. Your knees should be slightly bent. Bring your hands up toward the ceiling until you feel gentle tension in your shoulders and chest. See the illustration on facing page.

WARM UP AND COOL DOWN

It's important to warm up prior to exercising and cool down once you've finished. The warm-up allows your body to gradually adjust to

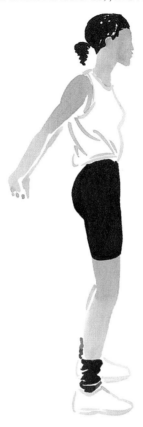

the vigorous workout you are about to perform, whereas the cool down allows your body to gradually return to its normal state. Note that the warm up I'm describing here is different from the brief warm-up you should do prior to stretching. Three to five minutes each for the warm-up and the cooldown is plenty.

Now, I know what you're thinking. It sounds like a lot to do. I'm asking you to warm up prior to stretching, stretch, warm up again, do your exercise, cool down, then stretch again. Well, it is a lot. But after a while, these other things will become part of your routine. They will give you time to mentally prepare, focus, and reflect on your workout. In time, you will see how it only enhances the experience of taking care of your body.

The best way to warm up and cool down is to use the same activity you are performing, only at a lower intensity. For example, if you are going to walk for 20 minutes, simply start out by walking at a slower, more comfortable pace for five minutes. Then, switch to a faster pace for your 20-minute workout. When you're done, cool down at the same pace you used for your warm-up. The same goes for jogging and stair stepping. Some step machines even build in a warm-up and cooldown in the pre-programmed routine. Most aerobic dance classes also include the warm-up and cooldown (as well as the stretching) in their typical 50- to 60-minute format.

Just another reminder: Stretching, the warm-up, and the cooldown do not count toward your 20 to 60 minutes exercise time. We'll talk about the amount of time you should exercise in Step Three. But now let's focus on how hard you should work.

Tips

► MAKE EXERCISE PART OF YOUR DAY—JUST LIKE BRUSHING YOUR TEETH.

► ARRANGE YOUR WORKOUT CLOTHES THE NIGHT BEFORE, MAYBE EVEN PLACE YOUR SHOES BY THE DOOR, SO THAT YOU ARE PREPARED AND MOTIVATED FIRST THING IN THE MORNING TO EXERCISE.

► EXERCISE WITH FRIENDS AND NEIGHBORS, MAYBE EVEN ARRANGE A WORKOUT GROUP. JUST BE SURE THAT YOU EXERCISE AT YOUR OWN PACE.

► FIND WAYS TO MAKE YOUR WORKOUTS MORE ENJOYABLE. LISTENING TO MUSIC IS A GREAT WAY. IF YOU WATCH TELEVISION OR READ WHILE YOU EXERCISE, JUST BE SURE TO MAINTAIN YOUR INTENSITY.

► AFTER YOUR WORKOUT, TREAT YOURSELF TO SOMETHING SPECIAL, SUCH AS A MASSAGE, BUBBLE BATH, MEDITATION SESSION, OR JUST LISTEN TO SOOTHING MUSIC.

Step Two

EXERCISE IN THE ZONE (AT A LEVEL SEVEN OR EIGHT)

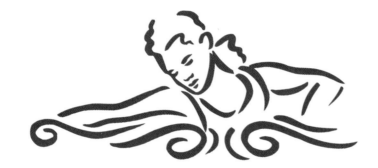

I used to think that showing up every day to work out was enough. It isn't. It's what you do and how hard you do it that makes the difference between losing weight and not. Working in the zone is the key to success. All of those times I'd start, then fail, a workout program, I would usually show up, but I would barely break a sweat. As a matter of fact, when I first started working out with Bob, I tried to explain to him how my body refused to sweat, and that I would be different from other clients he'd helped. I told him I could go for an hour and not sweat. "It's not only the length of time that you work out that heats up your body, but more important, the intensity at which you work out," he said. "Oh, no. It's my genes. I don't think I have a sweat gene!" I said. "Everybody sweats once they're trained and they work hard enough. You will too," he assured me.

Well, he was right. I need a beach towel now to soak up the sweat from my workouts. When you hit the zone, you sweat. And you sweat more the better shape you're in. And the better shape you're in, the more your body burns fat.

In my past exercise experiences, whenever I hit the zone, I'd stay there for a short while, then I'd prefer to work out at a slower pace. The success comes when you stick with it. It can be exhausting at first, but well worth the payoff. This is what I've learned—the harder you work, the easier it is to work hard.

—Oprah

A lot of people give up exercise because they don't see any results from it. They would exercise every day, perform the correct exercises, maybe even lose a little bit of weight. But eventually their weight would plateau and they could not reduce any further. This is very disheartening, especially when you are doing almost everything right. Don't give up on exercise. It is critical that you exercise in order to significantly change your metabolism. It is critical to exercise to be fit and free yourself from being overweight. So how can you exercise each day and still not lose much weight? By not exercising in the "zone." How long you exercise is important, but it is less important than how hard you exercise. If you are not exercising at the proper intensity level, no matter how long you work out, you will not see much weight loss. In fact, you may just break even. You won't gain any weight, but you won't lose any either.

One of the best examples of this was a client I worked with one summer. Don had been working out with a trainer for the past two years. He was actually fairly fit and ate a healthy diet, but he still had this extra ten pounds mostly around his midsection that he couldn't seem to lose. He and his trainer were not planning to work together that summer, and he invited me to their last workout to see what they were doing. He warmed up, stretched, lifted weights, walked on the treadmill for 45 minutes, and cooled down. All in all, a pretty good workout. Pretty good except that, while walking on the treadmill, he talked to his trainer, joked around, smiled, and laughed. He was hardly breathing above resting level, and I'm not sure I even saw a bead of sweat on his forehead. He was not working at the proper intensity. He was not in the zone!

In my first workout with him all that changed. I cut his exercise time down to 20 minutes and taught him how to rate the intensity of his workout. At the end of three weeks he was up to 30 minutes in the zone, and had lost eight pounds. At the end of four weeks, he had reached his goal weight. He's 42 and hasn't been at this weight since high school. He had his entire wardrobe altered.

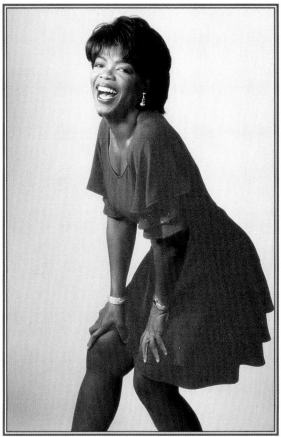

HARRY BENSON

Remember that it is possible for you to be doing all of the other nine steps correctly and not lose weight if your intensity is not high enough.

This is a crucial point for you to understand, and the information in this chapter is critical to your weight-loss process. I encourage you to read this chapter twice, if you don't understand it the first time. It involves learning a whole new skill.

This chapter and the next one are interrelated. Step Two has to do with the intensity with which you exercise. Step Three has to do with the amount of time you exercise.

IT'S ALL ABOUT INTENSITY

For many years, we were told in order to burn fat, you must exercise longer and slower. There are some people who still believe this. In part, that's because lab tests show that when you exercise at lower levels (50 to 70 percent of your maximum ability), you burn a higher percentage of stored fat versus stored carbohydrates. As you increase your intensity, you begin to burn a higher percentage of stored carbohydrates. This is true.

So, common sense might tell you that since it is fat that you want to burn, you should slow down your exercise to below 70 percent of your maximum ability. For those of us who don't prefer to exercise at slightly higher intensities—and that's just about all of us—this probably makes a lot of sense. But it's simply wrong.

The truth is, energy is energy. It doesn't much matter what fuel source you burn during your 20 to 60 minutes of exercise. What does matter is raising your metabolism for your 20 to 60 minutes of exercise and all the hours afterward. Low intensity exercise doesn't do much for your metabolism. But moderately high intensity exercise does. And when you increase your metabolism, you decrease your set point and your body fat.

Even the number of calories you burn during your exercise session becomes somewhat irrelevant. What's important is the rate you're burning calories both during your exercise session, as well as the other 23 1/2 hours of every day of your life!

Let me put it another way. How many golfers do you know who stroll on the golf course for four or five hours a day, three, four, or even five times a week? If they walk instead of ride in a golf cart, they are burning a large amount of calories each round. But I probably don't need to tell you that a lot of these same golfers can be lugging a spare tire around the middle. On the other hand, how many runners do you see carrying around that spare tire? Relatively few.

That's because you work harder when you're running than you

do when you're strolling the golf course. The intensity is higher. However, strolling the golf course for five hours will burn more calories than 30 minutes of jogging. Again, don't be fooled. Calories burned during your exercise session isn't what is most important. *Changing your metabolism is.* If you change your metabolism, you will change your weight.

Oprah was able to reach her goal weight through eating right and exercising. She used the steps that you are currently learning. When she first reached her goal weight, she did a show about it. At the time, she was running about eight-minute miles. (This does not mean that you will need to run eight-minute miles in order to achieve your goal weight!) This represented the intensity she needed to exercise at in order to maintain her weight. Then she decided to run the Marine Corps Marathon. But to do it, she had to train herself to run more miles. There was no way she could hold her pace of around eight-minute miles for these longer training runs. So she had to lower her intensity to 9.5-minute miles. She was surprised by what happened. Her weight began drifting up. Though it was only four or five pounds, the point was clear. Oprah had to exercise at a moderately high intensity level in order to lose or maintain her weight. Some days she would run more than three hours, but she never brought her intensity level back up to the point she needed to in order to lose those extra pounds. In other words, she was running longer, burning more total calories, but the rate that she was burning those calories was slower both during exercise and all of the other hours in the day. That's how she gained that little bit of extra weight, even while training for a marathon.

Keep in mind that Oprah ran a marathon to fulfill a personal goal. The extreme amount of exercise required to train for a marathon was not needed in order for her to lose weight. For her, exercising in the zone for 45 to 60 minutes a day, six or seven days a week, and following the other steps, allows her to maintain her desired weight. This is what it takes for her! For most people, less exercise is needed to achieve and maintain their goal weight.

FINDING THE ZONE: HEART RATE VS. THE SUBJECTIVE RATING SCALE

So, how do you find the zone? In other words, at what intensity should you exercise in order to change your metabolism? Exercise intensity has traditionally been expressed as a percentage of your maximum heart rate. I am going to continue expressing it this way so that it is easily understood, but I'm also going to show you a subjective way to gauge your exercise intensity because I feel this is the way most people should monitor their exercise intensity. I will be asking you to exercise at 70 to 80 percent of your maximum heart rate (seven or eight on the rating scale). To fully understand this, you will need the following information.

Your heart rate reflects the rate at which your body is using oxygen, as well as the rate at which it burns calories (metabolism). The more oxygen your body uses, the more calories you are burning. But remember, it's the rate you're burning the calories that's important, not so much the amount of calories you're burning. To estimate this rate of oxygen consumption, we often look at heart rate, or the number of heartbeats per minute.

If you have exercised before, you may already be familiar with the phrases "heart rate" and "target heart rate." Let me explain how we came to use heart rate to measure exercise intensity and some of the problems associated with this method.

Checking your heart rate during exercise is a fair way of measuring how hard you are working out. I consider it only a fair method because there are a number of other factors that can raise your heart rate, such as emotions, thoughts, lifting of heavy objects, the environment, even caffeine. In addition, you must stop exercising each time you want to know how hard you are working. Nonetheless, exercise professionals have traditionally used the heart rate to monitor exercise intensity. They give you a "target heart rate" based on a percentage of your maximum heart rate. Here's where the problems come in.

In order to get your target rate, you have to know what your maximum heart rate is. To get an accurate measurement of your maximum heart rate, you have to take a maximum treadmill test, in which you walk or run until you nearly drop. Sounds fun, huh?

To spare you the expense and inconvenience of the treadmill test, a formula (220 − your age) is used to estimate your maximum heart rate. To figure out your target heart rate, or the intensity level you should be working at, you have to take a percentage of your maximum heart rate. Usually this percentage is between 50 and 85 percent, depending on the philosophy of the person doing the prescribing.

Of course, I should point out, I believe nothing under 70 percent will produce the type of results we are looking for. Between 70 percent and 80 percent is what I call the " zone." This is the intensity at which I want you to learn to exercise. I also refer to it as the "results zone" because when you exercise consistently at this intensity, you get results. There may be times that you are unable to exercise within this zone. That's all right sometimes. When you exercise at an intensity of 60 to 70 percent, I call this the "maintenance zone." Below 60 percent I refer to as the "almost-wasting-your-time zone." There are some people who exercise between 80 and 90 percent. I don't recommend this for beginning or intermediate exercisers—it is more for highly trained athletes and is very difficult to maintain for your entire exercise session. Once again, when I refer to the "zone" I am talking about exercising between 70 and 80 percent of your maximum heart rate.

If you find all these numbers and equations confusing, you are not alone. Not only are they confusing, but they're also inaccurate. The equation that estimates your maximum heart rate is accurate for only a small percentage of the population.

Once you do figure out your target heart rate, trying to measure it during your workout can be next to impossible. Some of you know from aerobic dance classes how difficult it can be to pause during your workout, locate your pulse and count the number of heartbeats in ten seconds. An estimated 15 percent of all people can't even find their pulse—and I think that's a conservative estimate.

With all this confusion and difficulty in finding your heart rate, I want to suggest to you another method. First, I want to say there is no perfect way to monitor exercise intensity. But, I think what I am about to describe to you is the best way for most people.

A number of years ago, a scientist named Gunnar Borg developed a subjective scale to rate how hard you are exercising. The scale ranged from 6 to 20, and you rated how hard you thought you were working. His idea was basically good, but the numbers seemed to confuse people and his descriptions of what each number represented were somewhat vague.

Borg's scale was later modified using a range of 0 to 10. Using these numbers, you rate how hard you are exercising based on your feeling of fatigue. A rating of 0 would mean you are hardly working at all. A rating of 10 would mean all-out exhaustion.

I like this modified scale. I do, however, like to go into a little more detail about how you feel at each level, and have thus modified it a little myself. I think your breathing is one of the best indications of how hard you are working. So, for each number, I have given a detailed explanation of what you should be feeling and what your breathing should be like at each of the different levels.

I use this scale with all my clients, and it works. It may take you a little while to learn, but it's easy if you are aware of your body and what it's feeling. Among regular exercisers and highly trained athletes, you will probably notice that very few stop to take their pulse in order to figure out if they are working at their target heart rate. Instead, they become in tune with their bodies and instinctively know how hard they are working. You, too, can learn to feel how hard you're working.

Before I describe this scale, there are a couple of concerns I will mention. You may be in the ten percent of people who have a hard time subjectively rating your exercise. For you, it's difficult to feel how hard you are working. That's okay. Use the heart rate method. Then, there are some of you who may have certain medical problems that would be aggravated when you go above a certain heart rate. You will need to keep track of exactly what your heart rate is doing. Your physician can prescribe this heart rate for you. You may also use a combination of the two methods.

Now let's take a look at the scale and the level at which you should be exercising.

I want you to picture a scale from 0 to 10.

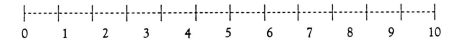

What you should be feeling at each level is listed below.

0. This is the feeling you get at rest. There is no feeling of fatigue. Your breathing is not at all elevated. You will not experience this at all during exercise.

1. This is the feeling you get working at your desk or reading. There is no feeling of fatigue. Your breathing is not elevated.

2. This is the feeling you might get while getting dressed. There is little or no feeling of fatigue. Your breathing is not elevated. You will rarely experience this low level while exercising.

3. This is the feeling you might get while slowly walking across the room to turn on the television. There is little feeling of fatigue. You may be slightly aware of your breathing, but it is slow and natural. You may experience this right in the beginning of an exercise session.

4. This is the feeling you might get while slowly walking outside. There is a very slight feeling of fatigue. Your breathing is slightly elevated but comfortable. You should experience this level during the initial stages of your warm-up.

5. This is the feeling you might get while walking briskly to the store. There is a slight feeling of fatigue. You are aware of your breathing and it is deeper than in level 4. You should experience this level at the end of your warm-up.

6. This is the feeling you might get when you are walking somewhere and are very late for an appointment. There is a general feeling of fatigue, but you know that you can maintain this level. Your breathing is somewhat deep and you are aware of it. You should experience this level in the transition from your warm-up to your exercise session and during the initial phase of learning how to work at level seven or eight.

7. This is the feeling you might get when you are exercising vigorously. There is a definite feeling of fatigue, but you are quite sure you can maintain this level for the rest of your exercise session. Your breathing is deep and you are definitely aware of it. You can carry on a conversation, but you would probably prefer not to. This is the baseline level of exercise that you will maintain in your exercise sessions.

8. This is the feeling you might get when you are exercising very vigorously. There is a very definite feeling of fatigue, and if you asked yourself if you could continue for the remainder of your exercise session, you think you could, but are not 100 percent sure. Your breathing is very deep, you can still carry on a conversation, but you don't feel like it. This becomes the feeling you should experience only after you are comfortable reaching a level seven and are ready for a more intense workout. This is the level that produces rapid results, but you must learn how to maintain it. Exercising at this level is difficult for many people.

9. This is a feeling that you would experience if you were exercising very, very vigorously. You would experience a very definite feeling of fatigue and if you asked yourself if you could continue for the remainder of your exercise session, you probably could not. Your breathing is very labored and it would be very difficult to carry on a conversation. This is a feeling you may experience for short periods when trying to achieve a level 8. This is a level that many athletes train at and it is difficult for them. You should not be experiencing a level 9 on a routine basis, and should slow down when you do.

10. You should not experience a level 10. This is the feeling you would experience with all-out exercise. This level cannot be maintained for very long, and there is no benefit in reaching it.

Take the time to learn each level. Remember, you are striving to achieve a level 7 or 8 during your exercise session. Level 7 equates to approximately 70 percent of your maximum heart rate, while level 8 equates to about 80 percent.

LEVEL SEVEN OR EIGHT

Everyone can exercise at a level seven. It may take you a while before you can sustain it for the minimum 20 minutes that I'm asking you to, but you will very quickly work up to it. Remember that when you first exercise at a level seven, you may not like the feeling. This usually goes away within the first month of consistently reaching a level seven. If you can't keep up a level seven, start at level six and step up to a seven for one or two minutes at a time. Keep extending the amount of time you do this until you are consistently working at a level seven. Usually within a week or two, every client I've worked with has been exercising at a level seven for at least 20 minutes. It may be a good idea to exercise with a qualified exercise professional for at least your first couple of sessions. I recommend that this person be certified by either the American College of Sports Medicine (ACSM) or the American Council on Exercise (ACE).

As I discussed earlier, when I first started in the field of exercise science, I was working with heart and pulmonary patients. These were people recovering from heart attacks and heart surgery. They had just been through one of the worst scares of their lives. And my job was to get them healthy and in shape.

A lot of people in my field believed that we should take it easy on these patients, that they should be exercising at much lower levels than everyone else. But watching these patients, I began to notice something. There were some who were comfortable working out at these lower levels and others who pushed themselves to work just a little bit harder. The ones who worked harder showed faster progress—they lost weight, got fit, began eating healthier, and stuck to the program I outlined for them. The ones who didn't work as hard saw fewer results, became frustrated, and sometimes dropped out of the program. Clearly, these heart patients were capable of exercising at moderate intensity levels—moderate for them. Perhaps it's walking to the mailbox when they first start out exercising. But to not push them to work within the zone is doing them a real disservice, because they will be doing little to change their condition.

The same point applies to people who want to improve their bodies and fitness level. When I began working with weight-loss clients, I noticed that the ones who worked just a little bit harder lost weight faster and had a higher rate of success overall. I also found when I increased the intensity of my own workouts, my fitness level improved significantly. If you push your body to do more, your body will respond by improving. But in pushing your body, safety is always the most important concern. I have spent a lot of time discussing why you should exercise at 70 percent and above. Also realize that at above 80 percent, you have limited additional gain and much more risk. So stay in the zone!

You may have already figured out that your level seven will be different from your friend's level seven, or your spouse's, or mine. That's why a heart patient can be working at a level seven and still get the same quality workout as a weight-loss client.

What's a level eight for Oprah is a level five for me. When I exercise with her—as I do with all my clients—I still have to do my own aerobic workout. One day after we had worked out, Oprah asked me to stop by her office. "Sure," I told her, "after my workout." She looked at me, surprised. "What do you mean? We just ran five miles." As politely as I could, I explained to her that the five miles we ran was at her pace and level of intensity. I still hadn't reached my intensity level for the day. Being as competitive as she is, she was slightly irritated. Then she went off to tape her show. After she left, I hopped on the stair stepper and worked out for 20 minutes at my level seven.

I maintained this routine even while training with Oprah for the marathon. There were days when we would run 10 or 15 miles. But always I would do an additional 20 to 30 minutes of exercise within my zone. That's because, in spite of the 10 or 15 miles I logged that day with her, I was working at her level seven and, therefore, was not doing enough to benefit my own level of fitness and my metabolism.

You will find that over time, the amount of exercise you can do at a level seven will change. Recall, that when Oprah first started walking, it would take her 17 minutes to complete a mile. That was while working at a level seven. As she became more fit and her body more conditioned, working at a level seven changed to jogging at a pace under nine minutes per mile. The level didn't change. What she could accomplish at that level did.

There are times you will want to change your level. If your weight plateaus, and you feel strong enough, you might want to work at a level eight for a few days a week. Or you might switch to an eight for a few minutes in your workout before returning to level seven. This is considered interval training. In other words, at different points in your workout, you work at a slightly higher level. If you are more advanced, you might try working briefly at an 8.5 or exercising at a level eight each day.

Now that you've got intensity down, let's focus on how long your workout should be.

Tips

▶ WHILE LEARNING TO RATE YOUR LEVEL OF EXERCISE, ASK YOURSELF FREQUENTLY, "HOW HARD AM I WORKING?" THIS WILL HELP YOU GET IN TUNE WITH YOUR BODY.

▶ IF YOU ARE NOT CAPABLE OF EXERCISING AT A LEVEL SEVEN FOR YOUR ENTIRE WORKOUT, START OUT AT A LEVEL SIX AND INCREASE TO A LEVEL SEVEN FOR ONE OR TWO MINUTES. AT EACH WORKOUT, ATTEMPT TO HOLD THAT LEVEL SEVEN JUST A LITTLE BIT LONGER. SOON YOU WILL BE ABLE TO DO YOUR ENTIRE SESSION AT LEVEL SEVEN.

▶ IF YOU ENJOY EXERCISING TO MUSIC, SELECT SOMETHING WITH A BEAT THAT MOTIVATES YOU TO EXERCISE AT A LEVEL SEVEN OR EIGHT.

▶ FREQUENTLY SET NEW PACE GOALS. IF YOU CONSISTENTLY WALK TWO MILES IN 30 MINUTES, TRY FOR 2.25 MILES IN THE SAME AMOUNT OF TIME.

▶ IF YOU WORK OUT WITH OTHERS, BE SURE TO EXERCISE AT YOUR OWN PACE. STRETCH AND WARM UP TOGETHER, BUT BE SURE TO EXERCISE WITHIN YOUR ZONE.

▶ YOUR MIND NEEDS TRAINING TOO. DURING YOUR WORKOUT, TRY FOCUSING ON SOMETHING OTHER THAN THE EXERCISE. FOR EXAMPLE, PRETEND YOU ARE WALKING THROUGH THE HILLS OF ITALY OR COMPETING IN AN ATHLETIC EVENT.

▶ IF YOU WALK OR JOG, HAVE A TIME TRIAL ONCE A WEEK OR ONCE A MONTH. TRY TO BETTER YOUR PERSONAL BEST TIME.

▶ TRY TO VIEW YOUR WORKOUT AS A MEDITATION SESSION. THIS HELPS SOME PEOPLE NOT TO FOCUS ON THE DISCOMFORT OF THE EXERCISE.

Step Three

EXERCISE FOR 20 TO 60 MINUTES EACH EXERCISE SESSION

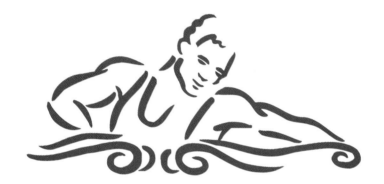

I have to be in the makeup chair with my hair washed and ready for blow drying by 7:30 A.M. in order to make a 9:00 A.M. show. Never would I have believed I could find time for exercise in my schedule—a schedule that is literally filled from the time I wake up until at least 8:00 P.M.. The only way to exercise consistently is to wake up every day an hour earlier. For me that means 5:00 A.M.. I'm proud to say that I've done it almost every day, without fail, for three consecutive years.

For someone like me, who could keep promises to everyone but myself, I consider this a major achievement. I used to view the exercise as such a chore. I don't anymore. I realized that on the few days that I missed a workout, I actually felt worse—and I don't mean from guilt. I was physically more sluggish, and not alert. The first time I realized this, I was leaving on a 6:30 A.M. flight to Arizona. I chose not to get up early to work out, thinking I'd make it up later in the day. I felt so tired and dull when I arrived, I asked for tea—the strongest they had—to help perk me up. It wasn't until late afternoon, when I forced myself into the gym for a thirty-minute burst on the treadmill, that I realized the very reason I was so tired and irritable was because I hadn't made time earlier in the day to crank up the furnace on my frozen metabolism. No matter where I am, and I've been in some remote places in the past three years, I now make time for the workout. I no longer even vacation in a place where I can't find a treadmill or a road I can walk or jog on. And on vacation it's the first thing I do when I wake up. I get at least 40 minutes out of the way so I can more fully enjoy the rest of my day.

Finding the time and making your workout the priority in taking care of yourself will determine whether you win for the long run. It's a life-giving process.

—Oprah

THE number-one excuse people make about not exercising is that they don't have the time. If you find yourself making all sorts of excuses about time, then you're not ready to make the commitment to exercise. And you're not ready to change your life.

Ask yourself: What is 20 or 30 minutes out of my day? It's about the same amount of time it takes you to watch a television show. In that time, you could be doing something good for your body and your life. And if you can't bear to miss your favorite show, then you can even exercise while you watch it.

And don't think you're too busy. That's a cop-out. Oprah has to be one of the busiest people I know. She usually tapes two shows a day, sometimes three, runs her own company, has dozens of meetings daily and travels frequently, yet she made room for exercise every day. And she is not alone. I have never met a client who could not build exercise into his or her day. But I've met plenty of people who didn't want to. I have a rule when meeting new clients: If they give me three objections to working out, I tell them I can't help them.

I think that just by reading this book, you have decided to do something to change your life. Now is the time for you to leave objections and excuses behind and go to work!

If you have not been active in quite some time, you might find it difficult to exercise for the minimum 20 minutes that is needed. If so, you will need to gradually work up to 20 minutes. Start by exercising for at least ten minutes. Then add a minute per week, until you are exercising for at least 20 minutes.

If you have no problem doing at least 20 minutes of continuous exercise, I recommend that you start working out for the minimum of 20 minutes. For some of you, this may mean a reduction in the usual amount of time that you exercise. That's all right. What is really important is that you exercise at the right intensity for those 20 minutes. I want you to work in the zone (level seven or eight). Get used to working out in the zone before you begin increasing the amount of time of your exercise session.

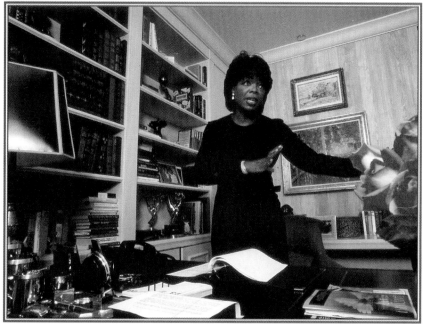

HARRY BENSON

Once you are exercising at the right intensity, for 20 minutes a session, 5 to 7 times a week, and following the other steps, your weight will likely decrease. But give it enough time. Remember how the physics of weight-loss works. You may hit a plateau now and then, so be patient.

As a rule of thumb, if you are faithfully following all ten steps, and your weight has either remained the same or increased over a three-week period, only then should you look at modifying any step. Step three is your best starting point, since you can simply add minutes to your exercise time until you begin dropping weight again. But make sure you are consistently following all ten steps before you begin adding minutes to this step. It may be that you need to exercise at a level eight at times in order to break through a plateau. But it's hard to figure that out if you aren't keeping up with the other steps. When you are comfortable exercising within the zone for the minimum of twenty minutes and feel you want to exercise longer, start by adding between two and five minutes to each workout session.

You may also be wondering how only 20 minutes of exercise a day can produce significant weight loss. Some of you may need more exercise time each day to get the results you want. Some of you will find 20 minutes will be plenty. Oprah must exercise at the right intensity for about forty minutes each day to maintain her weight. Again, that's because of her high set point. When I began working with Oprah, I was aware that she was used to quick results. So I had her work out for at least 60 minutes a day, usually split over two exercise sessions. Naturally, she got results more quickly. For most people, two workouts a day is not at all convenient. I would recommend you build up your exercise time within one session. And remember to be in the zone.

Soon after you begin exercising regularly, you will start to feel better physically and mentally. You will also get subtle signs that your metabolism is changing. Your clothes become looser, and you will have more energy throughout the day. At the same time, you will probably find that you are more tired by the end of the day. I mean a good kind of tired. You will also notice that you will sleep more soundly.

One of the best indicators that your metabolism is changing is in the way you perspire. When I first consult with someone, I always explain that it is important to work out long enough and hard enough to make you sweat. Virtually every time I mention this I get some version of, "I just don't sweat." The words may change. The way they're said may change. But I almost always hear those words. Trust me, you do sweat.

There are actually two reasons why people may not sweat when they exercise. First, when you're not active, your sweating mechanism goes into hibernation. You need to wake it up. Also, if you don't work out hard enough, even if you have been active, you probably won't sweat all that much. In other words, you are not in the zone.

I had scheduled an initial consultation with Susan. Susan was 36 years old and wanted to lose 18 pounds. This would put her at the weight she was at age 22. The week before we were supposed to have our consultation, I saw her at the health club that I belong to. She actually wound up on a stair machine next to mine. As we both worked out, she turned to me and said, "You really sweat." I answered, "Yeah, and you should be sweating too." Even before she replied, I knew what she was going to say. "I never sweat," she said. I told her to punch up her machine by two more dots. In two minutes, sweat was beginning to roll down her cheek.

The point is, we all sweat. You need to work hard enough and long enough to break a sweat. And, the better shape you are in, the more you sweat and the sooner you'll begin sweating in your workout. Now, Susan is jogging at a nine-minute-per-mile pace and is drenched within five minutes of her workout. She lost 16 pounds, which she says is all she wants to lose. In her words, "I look better than I did at twenty-two."

Now that you know how to exercise, let's focus on the other major component to getting fit: learning to eat right.

Tips

► IF YOU CHOOSE TO INCREASE YOUR EXERCISE TIME AFTER YOU HAVE IMPLEMENTED ALL TEN STEPS, ADD ONE OR TWO MINUTES TO YOUR SESSIONS EACH WEEK UNTIL YOU FEEL COMFORTABLE WITH THE AMOUNT. DO THIS ONLY WHEN YOU FEEL PHYSICALLY AND PSYCHOLOGICALLY READY.

► IF YOU WANT TO INCREASE YOUR EXERCISE TIME BUT HAVE ONLY LIMITED TIME IN THE MORNING, ADD A MINI-WORKOUT SESSION IN THE EVENING. THIS SHOULD BE A MINIMUM OF TEN MINUTES.

► TRY DOING YOUR PRIMARY EXERCISE FOR YOUR MINIMUM WORKOUT REQUIREMENT OF 20 MINUTES, AND FOLLOW IT WITH AT LEAST TEN MINUTES OF AN ALTERNATE EXERCISE.

► WHEN YOU HAVE THE TIME AND YOU FEEL READY, TRY DOING A LONGER WORKOUT SESSION (40 TO 60 MINUTES) ONCE A WEEK. SOON YOU'LL BE ABLE TO DO THIS TWICE A WEEK.

► REALIZE THAT A TYPICAL AEROBICS CLASS LASTS ABOUT AN HOUR, BUT THERE IS STRETCHING, A WARM-UP, AND A COOLDOWN WITHIN THAT ONE HOUR. THE ACTUAL AEROBIC PORTION IS USUALLY ABOUT 30 MINUTES, SO THAT IS WHAT IS COUNTED TOWARD THIS STEP.

► EVERY SO OFTEN, ARRANGE TO TEST YOUR ENDURANCE WITH A PERSONAL CHALLENGE SUCH AS A VERY LONG WALK OR JOG, OR ENTER AN ORGANIZED EVENT SUCH AS A 5-K OR 10-K WALK OR JOG OR A LONG-DISTANCE BIKE RIDE.

Step Four

EAT A LOW-FAT, BALANCED DIET EACH DAY

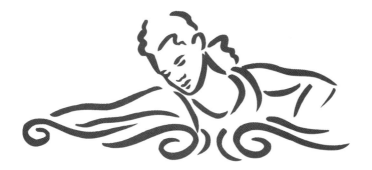

I used to crave potato chips. I ate them by the five-ounce bag. With 11 grams of fat per ounce, my two-day allotment of fat grams would go in one sitting. Recently I ate one ounce of the same fatty chips I used to scarf down by the pound and developed an upset stomach. I consider that progress.

For a girl like me, who grew up on fried everything—even vegetables simmered in fatback until every possible nutrient was drained or covered in grease—low-fat was a foreign concept. It was meeting Rosie and discovering that low-fat didn't have to mean low flavor, that helped me convert. Now, foods high in fat literally make me sick. Reducing the fat in your diet is a great step on the path to a healthier life. But just reducing fat for me wasn't enough to lose the excess pounds. For two years before I met Bob I ate only low-fat meals and snacks. Not only did I not lose weight, I gained. Partly because I never learned when to stop eating. I was a compulsive emotional eater.

For me the most difficult part of step four was learning to focus on what was troubling me. For you, the difficult part may be doing without the fat in your diet. This was also difficult for me, but in time I found that I no longer craved fat—it actually hides the real taste of foods. Just be patient, it doesn't happen overnight.

Reducing fat (sugar and salt as well) may at first jolt your taste buds. But in time, you too will prefer this healthier way of eating. And there is no question that you will feel better.

—**Oprah**

THIS step may be the most difficult behavior to incorporate into your life. Our eating habits are often ingrained over a period of years, and changing them might take years. But changing them is the only way to make a lasting difference in your life. Forget diets. They are only temporary solutions. Do not be confused by the word *diet,* which I use a lot in this chapter and the book. The word has come to be associated with a temporary way of eating adopted to lose weight. When I use the word, I'm really referring to the foods that you eat on a regular basis.

I'm asking you to change the way you eat: when you eat, what you eat, how you eat. I'm not concerned with every little thing you eat, nor am I telling you there are some things you should never eat. I'm concerned with the way you eat most of the time. If you stray every once in a while, fine. What's important is what you do consistently. The results lie in consistency, and that's true for all the steps.

I used to love pies. I still do. Less than ten years ago, I couldn't finish dinner without having a slice of pie. Lemon meringue. Pumpkin. Key lime. Pecan was my favorite. One day I decided I had to change, so I cut back, and now I have a slice maybe once a month. I almost never eat pecan pie. After cutting back I noticed I felt better, my exercise improved, and my cholesterol level—a problem in my family—dropped. I didn't completely cut pies out of my diet, I just stopped eating them all the time. Yet, it made a great difference to my overall fitness and the way I feel.

I would guess there are areas in all of our diets that we could stand to improve. The main point of this chapter is to learn how to get some of the fat out of your diet. In addition, I'm going to tell you how you can control how much you eat based on what your body requires. And finally I'm going to show you an easy way to make sure you are eating the right foods in the proper amounts. This chapter is loaded with lots of information. So get ready for a mini-course on how to establish a low-fat, well-balanced diet in your life.

TAKING OUT THE FAT

We actually need some fat in our diets. Fat helps in a variety of body functions, including assisting digestion, increasing our immunity to disease, transporting cholesterol, and making hormones. The problem is, most of us get way too much fat in our diets. You see, fat is a high-calorie nutrient. Fat contains more than double the amount of calories that you find in carbohydrates or protein.

Getting most of the fat out of your diet is essential for losing weight, as well as improving your overall health. High-fat diets contribute not only to our weight, but to cancer and heart disease. Our goal is to reduce the amount of total fat consumed in a day to between 20 and 50 grams.

All or most of the fat you eat should come from unsaturated fat sources such as olive oil, safflower oil, canola oil—oil from plant sources. The tropical oils, coconut and palm oil, come from plant sources but are exceptions. Butter, lard, coconut oil, palm oil, and the fat you find on animal meat are examples of saturated fat. They should essentially be eliminated from your diet.

I have given you a relatively wide range to work with here. If you consume 50 grams of fat, you are consuming two and a half times as much fat as someone who is eating 20 grams of fat. The reason I give you such a wide range is because we are all different. We all have different energy needs and different body chemistries. What works for one person does not necessarily work for another. This has been the downfall of many eating or weight-loss systems. They try to tell us what works for everyone.

But within all of the steps, I am asking you to find what works for you. For example, let's say you reduce your fat intake to 40 grams a day, and your weight drops, but it plateaus at a point well above your goal weight. After you review your performance on all of the other steps, you might decide to further reduce your fat intake to 35 grams. Your weight begins to drop again. What you discovered is that you can't go over 35 grams of fat each day in order to lose weight. You may need to reduce the amount of fat grams several times before you reach your goal weight.

Another example might be, you attempt to reduce the amount of fat in your diet from 30 grams to 20 grams, but you find it very difficult. You constantly crave foods that are high in fat. You never feel satisfied with your meals. And you notice that a particular side effect shows up, such as your skin becomes very dry. This is an indication to you that only 20 grams of fat each day does not work for you. You need to increase your fat intake. And you may have to modify one or more of the other steps in order to reach your goal weight.

Our bodies give us constant feedback. We just need to learn how to listen to them. As is the case with almost all of the steps, a little trial and error within the recommended ranges is a good idea.

You should start by reducing your fat intake to about 50 grams a day, unless you already consume less. For some of you this may represent a significant reduction in your total fat intake. If so, it may be difficult cutting back at first. I have known people who routinely consume over 200 fat grams a day. That's the amount of fat found in about 12 hamburgers. If you are consuming such excessive quantities of fat each day, any reduction is a positive step for your health. So, just gradually begin reducing your fat grams.

For all of you cutting back, you will likely find that you will crave fat for a while. That's because you are depriving your body of something it is used to having. These cravings will eventually go away.

When I first started working with Oprah, she had already been eating a fairly well-balanced, low-fat diet for about two years. Her fat intake was about 35 grams a day. To get more results, I reduced her daily fat intake to between 25 and 30 grams. Her weight began to drop immediately. But her cravings for fatty foods became more frequent. We would be talking about something totally unrelated to food, and Oprah would interject some statement like, "God, I haven't had a hamburger in I don't know how many years." Or once when we were talking about a trip to Maine, she broke out with, "Remember those fries they served in Nantucket?" This went on for about three months, around the time she was training for the half marathon in San Diego.

She made a deal with me that if she completed the half marathon, she would be allowed to go to one of her favorite restaurants and order whatever she pleased. I was all for it. She completed the event, and afterward we went to the restaurant. Once there, she ordered one of her favorite soups, smoked chicken, which was prepared with a cream base and loaded with fat. After about four spoonfuls, she decided she couldn't eat any more. The taste was just not the same. It was much too rich. That incident marked a departure for Oprah. She no longer required—and actually had a distaste for—foods high in fat. This is a common occurrence. It takes a little time, but once you become active and reduce the amount of fat in your diet, it will happen to you. Just be patient!

KEEPING TRACK OF FAT IN YOUR DIET

As long as you are consuming between 20 and 50 grams of fat each day, you are within the guidelines of this step. I'm not a big fan of having to count anything, but when you are learning about what to eat and how much, you will need to count fat grams for a while. I have found that usually within three months, most people no longer need to keep count. They are more aware of what to eat and quite naturally and automatically keep their fat consumption within the desired range.

In the meantime, it has become easier than ever to keep track of the amount of fat we eat. Food manufacturers have flooded the market with new, low-fat items. In addition, as you are probably aware, packaged foods now require labels that contain nutritional information,

Make the Connection

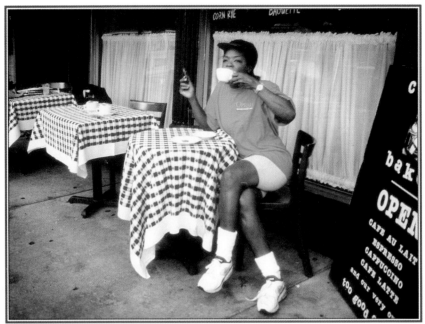

HARRY BENSON

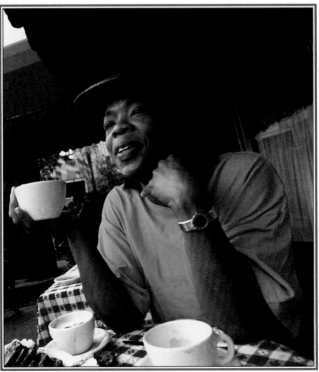

HARRY BENSON

including the fat content. You will find the fat content is expressed either in "calories from fat" or "grams of fat" or both. In one gram of fat there are nine calories. So it is fairly easy to convert calories from fat to grams of fat, if the latter is not stated on the package. Simply take the total calories from fat and divide by nine to figure out the fat grams. For convenience or to get information about foods that are not packaged or labeled, you can use a fat-gram chart. This chart lists hundreds of commonly eaten foods, and is available at your local bookstore or health food store. It's a good idea to have one.

DECIDING HOW MUCH FAT IS RIGHT FOR YOU

Again, it's up to you to decide, within the guidelines, how much fat to take out of your diet. Feel free to use a little trial and error. I recommend you start at the higher end of the range (40 to 50 grams a day), unless you are currently eating less. If you are already below 50 grams, I suggest you begin with cutting back by five grams a day. Adjust to this new level and see what your weight does. If your weight comes down, continue at this level. If you see no decrease, reduce the amount of daily fat grams by five more. Remember, too, there are other steps you can also modify. And give yourself enough time to lose weight, keeping in mind all the reasons that your weight can plateau.

It's better to reduce your fat intake more slowly and give your body time to adjust. In general, the less fat you consume, the healthier your diet. For most people, going below 20 grams a day provides little benefit and can actually cause health problems. The ultimate goal is to keep your fat intake between 20 and 35 grams each day. This may take one or two years to accomplish, and that's fine! Reducing the total amount of fat you consume can be an ongoing process. If you are a pregnant or lactating woman, you should consult your physician for recommended fat intake. Children and adolescents should also check with their physicians.

Keeping track of fat grams in your journal can be very helpful. The journal should be a resource of what works and what your body responds to. I'll cover this in more detail in step ten. Also, there may be some of you who like to keep an even more accurate record of fat grams by basing your fat intake on the number of calories you are consuming. For you, I recommend that 10 to 20 percent of your total calories come primarily from unsaturated fat. While this degree of accuracy is not essential, you can keep track this way if you prefer.

One last point about eating low-fat. With all of the new, low-fat products available, some nutrition experts are concerned that people mistake the low-fat label for permission to eat more. Some people are consuming the same or even more total calories and are somewhat defeating the purpose of eating low-fat. This has some truth to it. But if you know when to stop eating, this is not a problem.

WHEN TO STOP EATING

Now that you know how much fat you should be consuming, you probably want to know how much food you should eat. Keeping in mind what we discussed earlier about all the reasons we eat, understand that there are times we eat to satisfy what our bodies need and times we eat to satisfy something else. I'll go into more detail later about how to recognize the difference between the two.

How much food you eat, though, is an individual matter. Everyone is different, and the amount of food that is right for you would not be appropriate for someone else. The amount you should eat depends on your genetics, body size, gender, current metabolic rate, as well as a number of other factors. You can now understand why it's silly to put everyone on a fixed calorie diet and expect the same results.

The seemingly simple chore of eating the correct amount of food has been "packaged" and sold to us in so many ways I can hardly keep track. You can count calories, weigh all of your food, use food groups, consult one of many charts, or buy pre-packaged foods. You can even deal a meal. You have many options. But one thing I've learned through the years is, if you're not going to do it for life, it won't work. If you have to indefinitely rely on an eating system to know when to stop eating, you will not be successful! A system cannot take into consideration that, first, people are different, and second, each person changes his or her energy needs not only from year to year, but monthly, weekly, daily, and yes, even hourly! How can a system possibly keep up? It can't! But you can learn to recognize when you are eating to satisfy your hunger and when you are eating for other reasons.

What About Calories?

Your body expends a certain number of calories each day. Thinking, digesting food, your heart beating, walking to the refrigerator to get a snack, exercising, even moving your eyes while reading uses energy (calories). At the end of a day, you will have consumed a certain number of calories, and you will have expended a certain number of calories. If the number of calories you consumed is more than the number of calories you expended, your body stores the excess calories as fat. If the number of calories consumed is less than the number of calories expended, your body makes up the difference by diving into your fat stores for the needed energy. This all sounds so simple.

So why don't we just count the number of calories we eat and figure out how many we use and make sure we expend more than we consume? That has been the traditional method used to lose weight. The main problem with that simplified view of weight loss is that the rate of using calories (our metabolism) constantly changes, based on the amount and type of food we eat, the amount and intensity of activity we perform, as well as a myriad of other factors that continuously vary. This makes calculating the number of calories we expend virtually impossible.

There is a better way. Let's regulate our eating based on our current energy requirements. In other words, let's eat when we're hungry. This sounds so easy, but it is easier said than done for many of you. Weight problems usually arise when we eat past our hunger or cannot even recognize our hunger. It's a well-known fact that people who struggle with their weight have a hard time feeling their actual hunger. At the same time, active individuals tend to base their eating on their energy requirements to a much greater extent than inactive people. So, it seems logical that you should learn how to recognize when you're physiologically hungry and eat accordingly. That is what I'm going to teach you.

It takes a little time and effort, but this is very important. It will free you from a lifetime of counting calories. Let's not forget that you will be exercising at least five times each week. This, in itself, will enhance your ability to match your eating with your energy requirements. In addition, you should be keeping a journal during this learning phase, to help you uncover feelings about food, hunger, when and why you eat, and when and why you stop eating. Most important, you need to learn to recognize your hunger at each meal.

Your true hunger is a reflection of your nutritional needs—mainly your need for energy. Your goal is to meet those nutritional needs, but to stop just short of meeting your energy requirements. In other words, make sure you give your body enough nutrients, but don't eat until you're stuffed. In order for you to learn to feel your hunger, you need to experience being a little hungry. This means at the end of your meal, you should still want to eat—just a little. But that feeling will help you recognize your hunger. That slight feeling of hunger is your body warning you that it is going into your fat stores to make up the difference between calories expended and calories eaten. That's okay. This will reduce your fat stores. By performing this technique, you will learn to be hungry.

It's important to eat only when you're hungry. So, I want you to listen to your hunger prior to, as well as during, each meal. Listen for your hunger each time you eat a snack. Log in your journal why you began eating and what caused you to stop eating. Over time, you will learn to feel hungry. The goal is to eventually base all of your eating on your hunger and, thus, your body's energy requirements.

Oprah didn't learn to feel her hunger until recently. This is after spending her childhood and most of her adulthood eating for the wrong reasons. Four months after I began working with her, we were near the end of an eight-mile walk on the backroads of Indiana, when Oprah said, "God, I can't stop thinking about food." Nor could I. "I keep picturing food," I told her. Then I explained to her that our bodies were telling us that they were dipping into our fat stores. "In other words, we're hungry," I said. "What do you mean?" she asked. "You know, we're hungry. Haven't you ever felt hungry?" I said. Oprah hesitated. "Well, I'm starving now. And lunch isn't until one o'clock." That was at least two hours away. "Well, let's just move lunch up," I said. She gave me a look as if this was an impossibility since lunch was already scheduled. Her expression quickly changed when it dawned on her that we really could just change the time of lunch since we were hungry.

During that walk was one of the few times she had ever felt her hunger. Before then, she wasn't used to recognizing it. That's because at meals she always ate past her hunger, and in between meals, she always snacked so she never felt hungry. She ate for psychological reasons. She ate because of routine. She ate when she was tired, stressed, or just plain bored. She ate for every reason other than the most important one—because she was hungry. Having learned to recognize her hunger, she also learned that it's okay to eat when you feel hungry, even if it's not "time" to eat.

• • •

Psychological Hunger

For some of you, eating stops when you are satisfied psychologically, not physically. In fact, you may never reach that psychological satisfaction. That's because you're attempting to satisfy something else—something you may not even be conscious of—by using food. This psychological hunger should not be confused with physiological hunger. You need to learn the difference.

Any time you eat past the point of being hungry, ask yourself what you are thinking. Is something bothering you? Are you stressed out? You should write these thoughts in your journal. This will help you distinguish between physical and psychological hunger. It is a gradual learning process. But as you become more physically active, you will automatically improve your ability to eat based on your energy requirements, and reduce your psychological eating. You will improve even more by writing down your thoughts and feelings about when and why you eat, and keeping a record of instances when you eat for other reasons.

But you will likely need more immediate help in planning what and how much to eat. I don't think you should follow a system of eating forever, although it is helpful to refer to a system, not only for learning about energy requirements but other nutritional needs as well. You should use this system only until your body learns what its needs are. By then, you should be able to naturally make the right choices. I have found that the average person can do this within three months.

THE FOOD GUIDE PYRAMID

The system I like best is the Food Guide Pyramid. Realize that at some point in the near future, you will inherently know how much to eat at each meal. Some of you may already know. Nevertheless, I think this is useful information for everyone.

The Food Guide Pyramid was developed by the United States Department of Agriculture. It's an easy-to-follow plan that lists the types and amounts of foods you should consume daily. There are six basic food categories, along with recommended servings for each category (except the Fats and Sweets Group). This seems to be the simplest, most flexible system that I have found. And once you learn it, it's no longer a system. It becomes a natural way to eat. The pyramid is shown below.

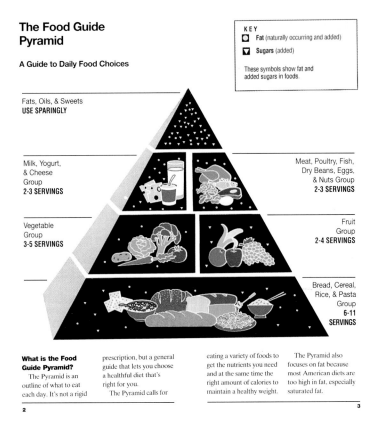

The Food Guide Pyramid

A Guide to Daily Food Choices

KEY

☐ Fat (naturally occurring and added)

☑ Sugars (added)

These symbols show fat and added sugars in foods.

Fats, Oils, & Sweets
USE SPARINGLY

Milk, Yogurt, & Cheese Group
2-3 SERVINGS

Meat, Poultry, Fish, Dry Beans, Eggs, & Nuts Group
2-3 SERVINGS

Vegetable Group
3-5 SERVINGS

Fruit Group
2-4 SERVINGS

Bread, Cereal, Rice, & Pasta Group
6-11 SERVINGS

What is the Food Guide Pyramid?
The Pyramid is an outline of what to eat each day. It's not a rigid prescription, but a general guide that lets you choose a healthful diet that's right for you.
The Pyramid calls for eating a variety of foods to get the nutrients you need and at the same time the right amount of calories to maintain a healthy weight. The Pyramid also focuses on fat because most American diets are too high in fat, especially saturated fat.

2

3

To use the pyramid, you need to eat within the guidelines of each food group. Keep in mind that the pyramid is a guideline. It is therefore important to find the number of servings within each group that is right for you, given your metabolism and your weight-loss goals. Some trial and error will probably be needed. If you are within the serving guidelines and not losing weight, you may need to decrease the number of servings from one or more of the groups. If you are at the minimum number of servings for each group and still not losing weight, you should look to one of the other steps to modify—a good choice would be step three (increase your exercise time). To review, each day you should have between:

6–11 Servings from the Breads, Pasta, Rice, Cereal Group

2–4 Servings from Fruits Group

3–5 Servings from Vegetables Group

2–3 Servings from the Meat, Poultry, Fish, Dry Beans, Eggs, and Nuts Group

2–3 servings from the Milk, Yogurt, Cheese Group

"Use sparingly" choices from the Fats and Sweets Group

Breads, Cereal, Rice, and Pasta Group (6-11 servings)

Sometimes I refer to this group as the whole-grains group, even though products made with refined flour are included here. The best choices in this group are always products derived from whole grains, such as whole-grain breads and cereals. More of their nutritional value is intact, and they contain more fiber. Also included in this group are pretzels and crackers. Pretzels make a great low-fat snack, but many crackers contain a lot of fat; be sure to read the label.

One serving equals:

1 slice of bread

$\frac{1}{2}$ cup of cooked cereal, rice, or pasta

1 ounce of breakfast cereal

1 ounce of pretzels (about one large Bavarian pretzel)

Fruit Group (2-4 servings)

This group includes all fresh fruit as well as canned and dried fruit. Fresh fruit is always preferred since it is loaded with vitamins, minerals, water, and fiber. Canned fruit should be eaten infrequently or not at all since it is usually packed in sugar. Dried fruits make a fair snack but should be eaten only occasionally, since they take up little space in your stomach and you tend to eat more of them. Eating fruit is actually part of Step Nine, and will be covered in more depth later.

One serving equals:

1 cup of strawberries, raspberries, blackberries, or boysenberries
1 medium-sized apple, orange, pear, peach, grapefruit, peach, or apricot
1 six-ounce glass of fruit juice
1 cup of cooked or canned fruit
1 banana
1 cup of grapes

Vegetable Group (3-5 servings)

This group includes all fresh, frozen, and canned vegetables. Fresh vegetables are always preferred to frozen and canned since they are higher in vitamins, minerals, water, and fiber. Frozen is better than canned. Make it a point to limit or eliminate the use of canned vegetables. Eating fresh vegetables is so important that I have made it part of Step Nine.

One serving equals:

$^{1}/_{2}$ cup of raw or cooked broccoli, corn, Brussels sprouts, green beans, or squash
6 ounces or $^{3}/_{4}$ cup of tomato or carrot juice
Lettuce, tomato, and onion (on a sandwich)
1 cup of leafy vegetables (as a base for a salad)

Meat, Poultry, Fish, Dry Beans, Eggs, and Nuts Group (2-4 servings)

I like to refer to this group as the high-quality protein group. Even though this group includes choices that can be high in fat and low in protein, you should select choices that are high in protein, low in fat. These choices include skinless chicken and turkey, lean cuts of beef, and occasionally pork. As for eggs, you should eat the egg white, as opposed to the entire egg, since virtually all of the fat and cholesterol is found in the yolk. Nuts are also part of this group, but they should be eaten on a very infrequent basis or not eaten at all because they are so high in fat.

One serving equals:

3 ounces of beef, chicken, or pork
1 cup of cooked beans (black beans, black-eyed peas, red beans, etc.)
3 ounces of cooked fish
3 eggs (remember to remove the yolks!)

Milk, Yogurt, and Cheese Group (2-3 servings)

This is a group in which you can trim away a lot of fat! You should have skim milk or 1 percent milk instead of 2 percent or whole milk, low-fat yogurt, and low-fat cheese or cottage cheese. You should choose frozen yogurt or sorbet over ice cream.

One serving equals:

8 ounces of milk
8 ounces of yogurt
1 ounce of cheese (this is natural cheese; processed cheese would be 2 ounces)
½ cup of cottage cheese

Fats, Oils, and Sweets Group

This group includes choices from all fats and oils such as canola oil, olive oil, palm oil, lard—any fat that you can cook with. It also includes sweets, such as cakes, pies, candy, pastries, and generally foods high in sugar content. You will notice that this group does not have a number of recommended servings. The less you eat from this group, the better. Since all of the fat you need is typically provided for by eating within the ranges of the other groups, the ideal number of servings from this group would be zero. For some people this may at first be difficult to achieve. If this is the case for you, gradually reduce the number of servings from this group until you reach the minimum number of servings you are willing to consume. Limiting servings from this group is one of the best things you can do for your weight-loss program and your overall health.

The food pyramid is an excellent guide to what makes a nutritious, well-balanced diet for most people. Again, since the Food Guide Pyramid was developed for people not necessarily looking to lose weight, I am going to suggest a couple of points specifically for those who are:

- Use fats in accordance with this step (20–50 grams/day).
- Milk should be skim or 1 percent.
- Yogurt and cheese should be low-fat.
- Meats should be lean cuts with excess fat trimmed off.
- Nuts should be avoided.
- You can have up to six vegetables a day.
- Two or even three fruits is best.
- Limit the servings of bread to one per meal.
- Sweets should be avoided or eliminated.

A FEW LAST WORDS ON EATING

Your meals exist to satisfy your energy requirements and meet your nutritional needs. They also exist for your enjoyment. Let's talk about enjoying each meal. You may be thinking you can only enjoy your meals based on what you eat or how much you eat. That is only part of it. Try shifting your focus to the company you share your meal with, the surroundings in which you have your meal, and the knowledge that you are eating something good for you. In short, focus on the eating experience.

To do this, you should make your meals an event. Plan to eat your meals in comfortable surroundings, invite interesting people to dine with you, play soothing music. This way you can take pleasure in more than just the food.

A number of years ago, I was given a tape of some classical music and decided to play it at dinner one night. I noticed that I was a lot more relaxed while eating. It became a habit to play relaxing music at dinnertime. Since I started doing this, I look forward to the dinner experience to a greater extent than ever before. I also did not want to ruin my appetite during the day so I could fully appreciate the whole experience. Conversely, after finally buying a television set, I once left it on during one of my meals. While watching a program, I found I ate faster without even enjoying what I was eating. It was as though all my excitement about my meal got zapped into the television screen. And afterward, I felt edgy and unsatisfied. The point is, make your meals a pleasant experience and enjoy them.

There are also places you shouldn't eat in your home and office. These are places that allow you to feel that it's acceptable to eat any-time—even when you're not hungry. I'm talking about eating in front of the television, in bed, at your desk, in the car. Take the time to enjoy the experience of eating—not only the food!

Here's one last point about food. There is not a food in existence that you can never eat. It is simply a matter of what food you eat on a regular basis and how much of it that dictates the success of your weight-loss program. If you fall off the healthy eating wagon, don't worry. Pick yourself up, and get right back to treating yourself well. Consistently performing all of the steps is the key to a new way of life!

Success with Step Four is simply a matter of taking the majority of fat out of your diet and knowing what to eat and when to stop eating it. Once you have learned what to eat, how much makes up a serving, and the appropriate number of servings for each food group, you will figure out, through trial and error, the amount of food needed for you to reach your goal weight and maintain it. I have never worked with anyone who did not become in tune with their body, given time and practice. The same will happen for you.

A Sample Day

Breakfast
1 ounce of packaged cereal (2 cups of shredded wheat)
8 ounces of skim or 1 percent milk
1 cup of strawberries
1 glass of grapefruit juice
Tea

Lunch
Turkey sandwich: 2 slices bread, 3 ounces of sliced turkey, lettuce, tomato, onion
1 cup of vegetable soup
6 ounces tomato juice

Snack
8 ounces of nonfat yogurt (sprinkle with wheat germ if desired)

Dinner

4 ounces of baked chicken breast

1 cup of brown rice

1 cup of broccoli

1 cup of corn

1 slice of French bread

Water with lemon

Snack

Pretzels (1 ounce)

Total servings

Bread, cereal, rice, pasta group	7
Fruit group	2
Vegetable group	5
Dairy	2
Meat, poultry, beans, eggs, nuts group	2

Tips

▶ AT EACH MEAL, GET INTO THE HABIT OF ASKING YOURSELF IF YOU ARE FULL OR SATISFIED.

▶ GRADUALLY PREPARE MEALS WITH LESS OIL UNTIL YOU NO LONGER NEED TO USE IT. EVEN UNSATURATED OILS SUCH AS OLIVE OIL ARE PURE FAT. CUT DOWN ON THE USE OF THEM ALSO.

▶ TRIM ALL VISIBLE FAT OFF MEAT AND POULTRY.

▶ SELECT LEAN CUTS OF MEATS AND POULTRY. AVOID FATTY CHOICES SUCH AS SPARE RIBS, BRISKET, SAUSAGE, BACON, DUCK, AND GOOSE, AND PROCESSED MEATS (BOLOGNA, SALAMI, ETC.).

▶ SELECT LOW-FAT FISH. LIMIT YOUR INTAKE OF HIGH-FAT FISH SUCH AS MACKEREL, RED SALMON, AND SARDINES. AVOID BUYING CANNED TUNA OR OTHER FISH PACKED IN OIL.

▶ MEATS, POULTRY, AND FISH AS WELL AS OTHER FOODS ARE BEST BROILED, BAKED, STEAMED, OR POACHED.

▶ AVOID FRIED AND GREASY FOODS.

▶ USE LOW-FAT SALAD DRESSING OR BALSAMIC VINEGAR ON YOUR SALADS.

▶ AVOID CREAM, CREAM SAUCES, AND GRAVY.

▶ LOW-FAT YOGURT SHOULD BE SUBSTITUTED FOR SOUR CREAM WHENEVER POSSIBLE.

▶ LIMIT YOUR BREAD SERVINGS TO ONLY ONE PER MEAL.

▶ WHEN EATING OUT, DON'T ALLOW THE BREAD BASKET ON THE TABLE BEFORE YOUR MEAL ARRIVES.

▶ IN PASTA DISHES, USE LESS PASTA AND MORE VEGETABLES.

▶ AVOID OR ELIMINATE HIGH-FAT DESSERTS SUCH AS CAKES, PIES, COOKIES, AND PASTRIES. CHOOSE FRUIT, SORBET, OR LOW-FAT FROZEN YOGURT.

▶ EAT LOW-FAT SNACKS. REPLACE POTATO CHIPS, CORN CHIPS, AND NUTS WITH PRETZELS, AIR-POPPED POPCORN, RICE CAKES, AND RAW VEGETABLES.

▶ TAKING THE FAT OUT OF YOUR DIET CAN BE AN ONGOING PROCESS. TURN THE PROCESS INTO A CHALLENGE. IT CAN EVEN BE FUN! MAKE THE REDUCTIONS OVER TIME.

▶ SELECT JUST ONE OF THE "BAD" FOODS THAT YOU FREQUENTLY EAT AND TAKE IT OUT OF YOUR DIET.

▶ REMEMBER THAT AS YOU BECOME MORE ACTIVE YOU WILL *NEED* TO EAT MORE. BUT GRADUALLY INCREASE THE AMOUNT OF FOOD YOU EAT AS YOUR METABOLISM INCREASES.

▶ SET REALISTIC GOALS FOR MAKING PERMANENT CHANGES. DO IT ON YOUR SCHEDULE. JUST COMMIT TO CONTINUALLY IMPROVING THE WAY YOU EAT.

▶ TRY HERBAL TEA DURING MEALS AND AS A SNACK

▶ REPLACE MAYONNAISE WITH MUSTARD.

▶ STEAM VEGETABLES WITH CHICKEN BROTH AS OPPOSED TO PLAIN WATER.

▶ USE SALSA AS AN ALTERNATIVE TO HIGH-FAT CONDIMENTS AND DIPS.

Step Five

EAT THREE MEALS AND TWO SNACKS EACH DAY

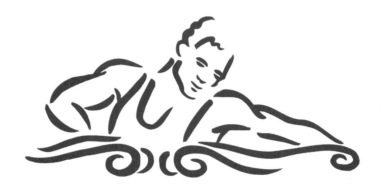

S ating increases your metabolism. Isn't that great news! When Bob first told me this my response was, "Then why don't I have the best metabolism on the planet?" I learned that the key is what you eat, how much you eat, and how often you eat. Three meals and two snacks spread throughout the day, with the greater proportion of calories eaten early in the day, will help you tremendously in controlling your weight.

I know this to be true. I've proven it over the past three years. But this is still the hardest step for me. Like most people, I've been programmed over the years to eat the biggest meal at dinner. Dinner should either be equal to or less than your other two meals with respect to calories, volume, and fat content.

I've learned that when I eat smaller meals throughout the day, I'm less hungry and I get the added benefit of keeping the flame under that metabolism of mine. When you eat this way you never get that stuffed, let-me-roll-onto-the-sofa, Thanksgiving feeling. You're burning calories more efficiently. Your body is also more grateful and will reward you for it.

—**Oprah**

JOANNE had been trying to lose seven pounds for about two years. She came to me because she believed there was something else she should be doing. As I listened to her describe her workout routine, I was amazed at her knowledge regarding exercise. She also had her diet

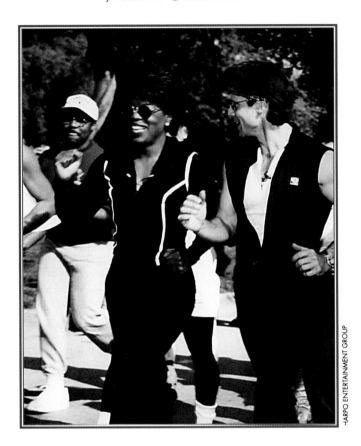

down pat. The only problem I could see was the distribution of food throughout the day. Joanne ate a very small breakfast, a snack between breakfast and lunch, a small lunch, and a relatively large dinner—much like the traditional American diet.

The first change I made in her diet was to add a snack between lunch and dinner. Next, I wanted her to decrease the size of her dinner by about 200 calories and redistribute those calories equally between breakfast and lunch. The end result was she would be eating more total calories with the addition of the snack, but consuming those calories earlier in the day.

Nine weeks later, Joanne had lost eight pounds. And she

couldn't believe she'd lost them by simply changing when she consumed her calories.

Wouldn't it be great if we all responded so easily to such slight diet modifications? This was Joanne's last step to reaching her goal weight. She was doing everything else correctly. And in her metabolism chain, this was the last link that needed to be strengthened. This practice can help you too. But first you need to understand it.

Eating increases your metabolism. You can actually eat more, within reason, and lose weight. We've already talked about what you should eat and how much. Now let's talk about when you should eat.

By eating three meals—breakfast, lunch, and dinner—and two snacks, you will be spreading your calories throughout the day. Don't fall into the trap of believing that by depriving yourself of food, you will lose weight. This is not true. On the contrary, withholding food will actually work against you. Your metabolism needs food to keep it elevated. When your metabolism is deprived, such as when you're on a low-calorie diet, it responds by shutting down.

You need to eat. And you need to eat more frequently. If you eat just one large meal a day, you will give your metabolism one little boost. But for the rest of the day, your metabolism receives little help. When you spread your eating throughout the day, you give your metabolism a boost at each meal and snack.

Let me give you an example. Let's say you decide to skip breakfast and lunch, omit all snacks, and eat a 1,600-calorie dinner. Your metabolism would get a boost at dinner time, and that's all. In addition, when you consume large quantities of food at one sitting, your body produces extra insulin. This takes the excess calories your body doesn't use and converts them into fat. Not at all what you want.

Compare that day with taking the same 1,600 calories and spreading them among three meals and two snacks. Your metabolism receives a boost each time you have a meal. That means it's working harder all day. And you do not have the corresponding insulin effect that you get by eating one large meal. The net result is, by spreading your meals throughout the day, you do not send a signal to your body to deposit fat. Eating one or just a couple of meals a day tells your body to store fat. The message is simple: Eat three meals and two snacks each day!

Some of you, like Oprah and myself, will need to eat a little something before you work out. Remember you will be exercising first thing in the morning. I'm not saying you should work out on a full stomach. I'm just telling you that you might find, as you increase the time and intensity of your workouts, you need to eat a snack before you exercise. Some of you will prefer not to eat anything. Should you choose to do so, you won't need to count this pre-exercise food as one of your meals or snacks. In effect, it becomes an optional third snack. If you have this snack, eat it soon after you wake up, so that by the time you dress for your workout and stretch, your body will be ready to exercise. Your snack might be some fruit, an English muffin (or half), or perhaps some fruit juice. You'll know what you crave.

I started this chapter with the example of Joanne to impress on you how important it is to eat more of your calories early in the day. This will elevate your metabolism over and above its usual incline. Recall that your metabolism starts out slow in the morning and gradually rises to its peak around dinner time. To have the greatest impact on your metabolism, you want to boost it when it's at its lowest, which is earlier in the day.

It's interesting to note that we traditionally have a small breakfast, or skip it altogether, a somewhat larger lunch, and by far our largest meal at dinner. To add insult to injury, we then do most of our power snacking late at night. This equates to the best plan for packing on the most pounds! What we should be doing is eating a solid breakfast, a solid lunch, two or three snacks, and a smaller dinner. In fact, in the ideal day, each meal would consist of about the same amount of calories, and the snacks would be about 80 to 150 calories each. Some ideas on what to eat for meals:

Breakfast:

Three egg-white omelet filled with vegetables, or

Low-sugar cereal (shredded wheat, bran, etc.) with skim or 1 percent milk, or

Oatmeal or cream of wheat (with or without fruit)

Lunch:

Lean turkey or chicken sandwich and (non–cream base) soup, or

Salad (low- or no-fat dressing) with chicken, turkey, or fish and soup, or

Turkey, chicken, or fish and brown rice and vegetables

Dinner:

Pasta with vegetables, or

Pasta with chicken or fish, or

Chicken, turkey, or fish with two vegetables and brown rice, or

Three egg-white omelet with 8- to 10-ounce potato and vegetables

Some ideas for snacks:

Vegetables (raw or cooked, without butter)

Fruits

1 ounce pretzels

Low-fat frozen fruit or yogurt bars

Air-popped popcorn (season with Tabasco, vinegar, or cayenne pepper)

Rice cakes

Low-fat cookies

Soup (non–cream base)

Baked potato (without butter or sour cream)

Brown rice (without butter)

$\mathcal{T}ips$

- ALWAYS SIT DOWN, PREFERABLY AT YOUR KITCHEN OR DINING ROOM TABLE, WHEN YOU EAT.

- AVOID EATING AT YOUR DESK.

- MAKE EACH MEAL AND SNACK AN EVENT: PLAY MUSIC, INVITE INTERESTING PEOPLE OVER, EAT IN A PLEASANT, RELAXED ENVIRONMENT.

- LIMIT THE AMOUNT OF TIMES YOU EAT OUT IN THE BEGINNING OF YOUR PROGRAM.

- LIMIT SOCIAL OBLIGATIONS THAT YOU KNOW INVOLVE FOOD THAT IS NOT HEALTHY. PEOPLE REALLY WON'T BE OFFENDED IF THEY CARE ABOUT YOU.

- ACTIVELY LOOK FOR NEW LOW-FAT MEALS AND SNACK IDEAS. SHARE THESE IDEAS WITH YOUR FRIENDS.

- KEEP YOUR SNACKS TO BETWEEN 80 AND 150 CALORIES.

- TRY SNACKS WITH DIFFERENT TEXTURES FOR A CHANGE OF PACE.

- ARRANGE TO HAVE MEALS WITH OTHERS WHO ARE COMMITTED TO EATING HEALTHIER.

- PLAN VACATIONS AND BUSINESS TRAVEL AT HEALTH-ORIENTED HOTELS OR SPAS. WHEN POSSIBLE, CHOOSE DESTINATIONS THAT ARE NOT RENOWNED FOR SERVING EXCESSIVE AMOUNTS OF FOOD.

Step Six

LIMIT OR ELIMINATE ALCOHOL

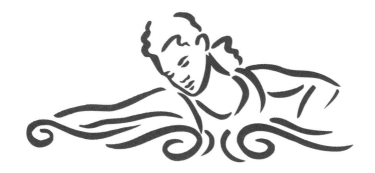

I was visiting Italy with some friends in the summer of 1994—the summer before I ran the marathon. One of the friends was Alan Richman, special food and wine correspondent for GQ magazine.

This was heaven for me, traveling with Alan, who knew all the best places to eat, in a place I think is the best place to eat in the world—Italy! Every night was a culinary feast. From Milan to the small towns of Umbria, we ate fresh-baked foccacia, seafood, pizza, pastas, risotto, you name it, we had it. We drank delicious wine every night. I made a deal with Bob: Just let me eat and drink what I want this one week. Then I won't have another drink until after the race. I'll exercise twice as hard. I'll stay in the zone every workout. I won't let the wine affect my workout. It's my vacation, for goodness sakes! I'm supposed to have wine if I want it. So we made a pact. Our running workouts would continue as usual. We were four and a half months from the marathon.

Bob had warned that there was no way I could drink much alcohol and maintain my strength. I was determined to prove him wrong. We had a great feast at a castle in Umbria one night—with the best wines from the Antinori vineyard. It was a glorious meal.

The next day started out equally glorious. The sky was so blue, it looked like a painting. There were only a few clouds scattered over the rolling hills of Umbria—hills that, when you looked afar, had patchwork designs that seemed to never end. In the distance I could see a quaint little church with a steeple. "How beautiful! Let's run to that church and back." I said to Bob. "That looks like about a seven-mile run."

I was determined. Focused. Ready to make this a run to remember, determined not to let last night's wine have an impact on me at all. Focused on leaning into the hills, breathing, finding my pace, and holding it. The first minute I was breathing hard—what was wrong with me? "I just need

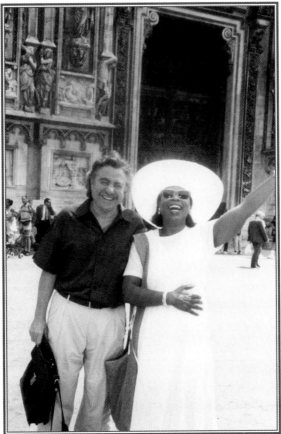

OPRAH WINFREY COLLECTION

to concentrate," I thought. "Concentrate, pick up my feet, breathe—
you're just getting started. Seven miles is a while—get movin', girl! Maybe
I should sing. 'She'll be comin round the mountain when she comes'—
nope, that won't work, can't sing and breathe, not enough oxygen. What's
the altitude here, anyway? Why do I feel like there's a wall in front of me
that I can't break through? My feet feel like lead. Or is it my thighs—no,
it's my whole leg!"

Both my legs are two lead poles that don't want to move. Five minutes
into the run, I still can't get my breathing regulated. Ten minutes and I still

can't find my rhythm. I so wanted to enjoy this run; the scenery was like a postcard.

Up ahead I hear Bob yelling, "Remember your word!" Yea, yea, yea, I remember, I say to myself. Can't you see I'm struggling here? I don't care if I never see that church with the steeple. Up close it probably looks like every other church I ever saw.

At the top of the hill, Bob calls down to me and says, "This is when you pay for that Montrachet." "So now he's a poet too," I said to no one in particular. He was beginning to get on my one last nerve. I was frustrated mainly with myself. When he said come on, you can do it, I did something I'd never done before. I shot him a bird. Yes, I gave Bob the finger.

I stopped running, and walked the rest of the way. It was difficult even walking up those hills. How much wine did I have? Just enough to be social. Three or four glasses, tops. Needless to say, the wine made a liar out of me. My body just wouldn't perform as I knew it could. I learned from that experience how alcohol adversely affects a workout, not to mention the rest of your day. You're just not as sharp. That's why it's called a depressant. It took me three days to feel like I could do a normal workout.

That may vary for you, but just know this—alcohol slows you down, and you may not even be conscious of it. Working out just allows you to be more aware of this.

—**Oprah**

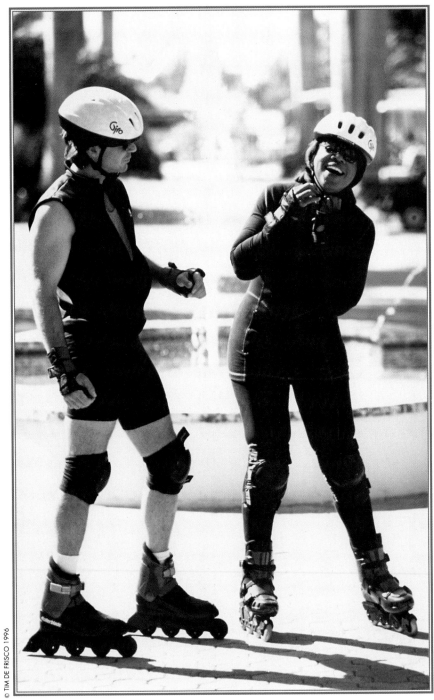

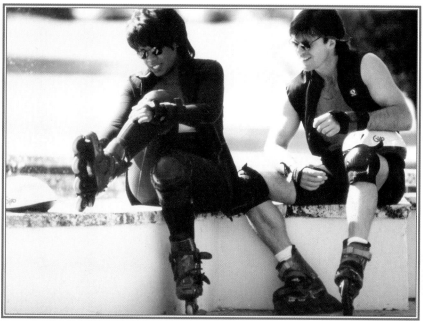

© TIM DE FRISCO 1996

I never really drank that much alcohol. But every now and again, I can appreciate a cool glass of chardonnay on a sunny afternoon. I also enjoy a good red wine with a pasta dinner. Every so often, I daydream of a cold beer on a hot summer day. So when I ask you to give up or at least limit alcoholic beverages, understand that I've had to do the same thing myself.

Although I had studied the effects alcohol has on the body, it wasn't until I lived at a high altitude that I really understood them. The apartment I rented in Telluride, Colorado, was right off the ski slope at just about 9,800 feet above sea level. My second week in town, I met some friends at a local pub. I had one beer. The next morning, I felt terrible. I was fully aware that the altitude can have funny effects on you. I was also aware that alcohol consumed at high altitudes has about triple the effect of alcohol consumed at sea level. But one beer?

About a month later, I toasted the opening of the spa where I worked with a glass of wine. The next morning I again felt terrible. It had to be the alcohol. This effect just goes with the territory. So, I gave up alcohol for a while. It was simply not worth the price. But by giving up alcohol, I also discovered that I felt better overall. It's easy to see how this is true if you live at high altitudes. It's not as easy to grasp at lower altitudes. But alcohol does affect you, no matter how subtle its impact.

Alcohol has too many strikes against it when it comes to losing or maintaining your weight. First, alcohol is quite high in calories. Compared to other energy sources, alcohol is only slightly better than pure fat. This is illustrated below:

Carbohydrates	= 4 calories per gram
Protein	= 4 calories per gram
Alcohol	= 7 calories per gram
Fat	= 9 calories per gram

The second strike against alcohol is that it is absorbed from the stomach into the bloodstream almost immediately, which means that it does not have a filling effect on you. So in addition you fill up on food, and that further increases the total calories you consume.

And worst of all, alcohol slows your metabolism. It is a depressant. So, after the big New Year's celebration, your metabolism limps along until January 4th!

If three strikes aren't enough, alcohol also has a lasting effect on your willingness and ability to have intense, quality workouts. Oprah recently had a few people over to celebrate her 42nd birthday. She turned to me and said, "Yes, Bob, I'm forty-two today, and I'm having some champagne." I said, "Great, where's mine?" We each toasted her birthday with one glass. The next morning we met in the gym. We were each on a stair stepper when Oprah looked at me and said, "This feels really hard today." It was unusual for me to agree, but I said, "I know." For the next ten minutes, neither of us said anything. Then midway through our workout, we both turned to each other and, at the same time, said, "Champagne." It was the glass of champagne the night before that was making our workout so difficult.

This effect can actually linger for days after overindulging. And, when you drink alcohol, you are much more willing, and likely, to abandon your program of healthy eating. You tend to adopt a "who cares" attitude—at least until the alcohol wears off.

For all of those reasons, if you can eliminate alcohol altogether, do so. If you are not willing to eliminate it entirely, I recommend you at least cut your consumption in half. Simply, estimate what you drink weekly and divide it by two. For example, if you are accustomed to consuming eight alcoholic beverages a week, your new alcohol budget is four per week. The good news is, when you begin to cut back, you are less willing to imbibe, since you feel alcohol's ill effects to an ever greater extent.

Most important, remember the more you restrict your alcohol consumption, the greater your long-term weight-loss results will be.

Tips

- THE FIRST DRINK USUALLY TASTES THE BEST. IF YOU PAUSE TO THINK ABOUT IT, THE SUBSEQUENT DRINKS ARE NOT WORTH THE DAMAGE!

- FILL UP ON WATER AND VEGETABLES PRIOR TO ATTENDING A SOCIAL EVENT WHERE ALCOHOL WILL BE SERVED.

- USE LESS ALCOHOL WITH EACH DRINK. FOR EXAMPLE, IF YOU ARE DRINKING WINE, CUT IT WITH SPARKLING WATER TO MAKE A SPRITZER.

- DON'T FEEL SOCIAL PRESSURE TO DRINK. IF YOU FEEL YOU NEED A GLASS TO HOLD DURING A PARTY, TRY A SUBSTITUTE. CLUB SODA OR SPARKLING WATER WITH LEMON OR LIME ARE GOOD ALTERNATIVES.

- CONSIDER ALTERNATIVE PRODUCTS SUCH AS NONALCOHOLIC DRINKS OR NONALCOHOLIC BEER.

- REALIZE YOU CAN HAVE AN APPRECIATION FOR FINE WINES AND BEER, BUT YOU DO NOT HAVE TO OVERINDULGE.

- BREAK THE ASSOCIATION BETWEEN DRINKING ALCOHOL AND HAVING A GOOD TIME. COMMIT TO REDUCING YOUR ALCOHOL CONSUMPTION BY A CERTAIN PERCENTAGE EACH MONTH.

Step Seven

STOP EATING TWO TO THREE HOURS

BEFORE BEDTIME

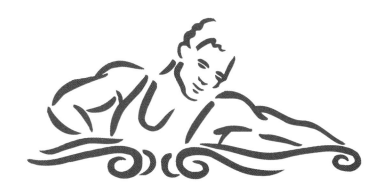

*Y*ou've no doubt heard the expression "Just do it." Well, when it comes to this step, that's my advice. Just do it. Stop eating two to three hours before bedtime. Don't question it, or try to get by with only one hour before bedtime. Don't even get out of bed and go into the kitchen for the famous midnight snack. Don't do it!

Just a little something before you go to bed lies around in your belly while you sleep. Picture that pretty sight. Picture it still lying there in the morning. Worse yet, picture it hanging on your thighs or your midsection 'cause it had no way to burn itself off. Get the picture?

Well, I gotta tell you, I learned early while working with Bob what a difference following this step made on my body weight. On weeks when I followed it, I could count on a two- to two-and-a-half-pound weight loss. If I cheated on this step, it sometimes meant the difference between dropping extra pounds or gaining. So now when I go to bed feeling like I could eat just a little something, I don't go grazing through the cabinets. I consider such a craving a good feeling. It means my body is dipping into my fat stores and burning the fat. And you know, I sleep better too!

—Oprah

GROWING up, I always had something to eat before bedtime. Milk and cookies, hot chocolate, ice cream, maybe even a piece of pie. Mom, Dad, my sister, and I would meet, usually in our pajamas, in either the kitchen or the family room just before bedtime. I always looked forward to it. Plus, there was always the unspoken notion that you would sleep better—especially if the snack included milk—as

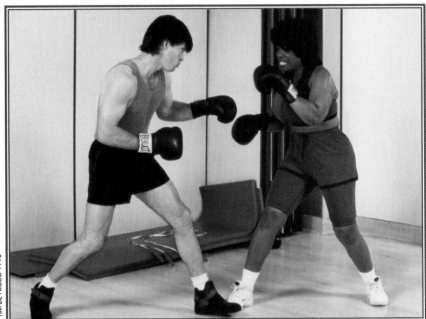

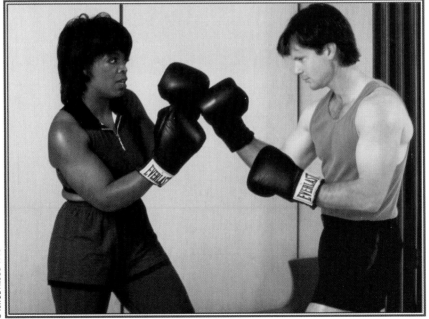

© TIM DE FRISCO 1996

© TIM DE FRISCO 1996

long as you didn't eat too much. I tell you, once I learned that this little late-night treat was not very good for me, the thought of giving it up was tough. So I didn't. I simply make it a healthy snack and eat it two to three hours *before* bedtime. Hey, some things are sacred!

This step comes down to planning. In general, the earlier you eat your meals, the better. The sooner you finish eating for the day, the better.

As we talked about earlier, your body's metabolism changes slightly throughout the day. In the morning it is relatively slow. As your day goes on, your metabolism increases, until it peaks in the evening. When you sleep, your metabolism decreases to its slowest level, until just before you wake up. Then the entire cycle starts all over again.

You also learned that both eating and exercising act to increase your metabolism. Again, I recommend that you exercise in the morning, in part because it revs up your metabolism early in the day so that you burn a higher rate of calories all day long. In addition, I talked about how important it is to move more of your calories toward breakfast and lunch and away from dinner, again to rev up your metabolism early in the day.

You might ask then why you can't also add calories at dinner and bedtime to further boost your metabolism. It appears that in response to eating, your metabolism does not increase to the same extent late in the day. So, in effect, calories eaten late in the day are just kind of waiting around to be converted to fat. It's almost as if your body knows that sleep is inevitable and it does not want to be "revved up." And as you know, once you do fall asleep, your metabolism plummets regardless of what you've eaten. This effect is not fully understood. But, in theory, your body reaches a metabolic maximum late in the day—perhaps to prepare for impending sleep. So calories eaten late in the day or, worse, around bedtime will be converted to fat more quickly.

We are working in theory here, since metabolism is hard to measure accurately. Though you cannot measure the small changes in your metabolism that will happen with each step you incorporate into your daily routine, realize that these changes will result in a relatively large difference in your weight over time. It's critical that you understand this, because to be successful at long-term weight loss, you must be both consistent and patient!

I have noticed through the years that clients who are able to stop eating two to three hours before bedtime are much more successful at losing weight and keeping it off than those who eat later at night and at bedtime. With most of these clients, it was a challenge at first to eliminate late-night eating.

The best example I have is myself. I have been very active all my life and have not had great struggles with my weight. But when I first started eliminating my late-evening eating, I immediately dropped three pounds. That's a lot for me! This is three pounds that never comes back unless I start eating within two hours of bedtime.

The key for those who are successful at long-term weight loss has been to effectively plan their meals and snacks and to overcome the urge to eat late at night. When you have that little craving for food in the evening, visualize your body going into your fat stores to satisfy your need for energy. In the beginning you will want to give in to that feeling. But in time, you will understand that the feeling is your body losing fat!

As for planning your meals and snacks, I have outlined below an example of a typical eating plan. You can modify this plan to fit your schedule.

A sample day based on a 6:45 wake-up time:

6:45 A.M.	Wake up
7:00 A.M.	Pre-workout snack
7:15 A.M.	Stretch, warm up
7:30 A.M.	20 minutes of walking, ten minutes cool down, and stretching
8:10 A.M.	Shower
8:30 A.M.	Breakfast

Noon	Lunch
3:00 P.M.	Snack
6:00 P.M.	Dinner
8:00 P.M.	Snack
10–11:00 P.M.	Bedtime

This may require you to change your current habits, but remember that's what this book is all about. You can experiment with different eating plans regarding your meals and snacks, and eventually you will come up with the perfect system for you. Just remember not to eat two to three hours before bedtime! You'll not only sleep better and feel better, you'll be helping yourself lose weight as well.

Tips

▶ THE KEY IS TO PLAN YOUR MEALS EFFECTIVELY. DO NOT SIMPLY MOVE YOUR BEDTIME BACK BECAUSE YOU ATE SOMETHING TOO LATE. MOVE YOUR MEALS EARLIER, AND OVER TIME YOU WILL NOT CRAVE FOOD LATE AT NIGHT.

▶ THINK ABOUT HOW EATING LATE AT NIGHT IS OUTSIDE YOUR BEST INTEREST AND CAN CAUSE YOU UNWANTED POUNDS. THIS CAN HELP YOU THROUGH EVENINGS OF TEMPTATION.

▶ A CRITICAL ASPECT OF THIS STEP IS TO EAT BREAKFAST AND EAT IT EARLY. YOU MIGHT NOT BE HUNGRY WHEN YOU FIRST START DOING THIS, BUT THAT WILL CHANGE AFTER YOU ARE USED TO EATING FIRST THING IN THE MORNING. EATING AN EARLY BREAKFAST TAKES THE EDGE OFF YOUR HUNGER THROUGHOUT THE DAY, INCLUDING AT BEDTIME.

▶ PLAN TO DO OTHER THINGS BESIDES EATING, SO THAT YOU AREN'T RESTLESS AT NIGHT. READ A BOOK, WATCH A FAVORITE SHOW, TAKE A BATH, OR LISTEN TO SOOTHING MUSIC.

▶ COMMIT TO EATING BREAKFAST. THIS TENDS TO DULL YOUR APPETITE IN THE EVENING HOURS.

Step Eight

DRINK SIX TO EIGHT GLASSES OF
WATER EACH DAY

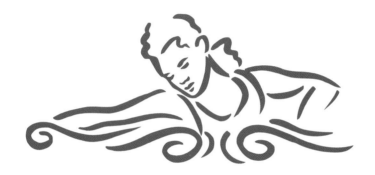

I've tried water plain out of the tap, bottled sparkling, bottled without carbonation. With a slice of lime, a slice of lemon, or an orange wedge. I've had it flavored with cherry, raspberry, peach, and wild berry, whatever that is! I've had it right out of the bottle, in small glasses, large glasses, plain glasses, and fancy glasses. And the bottom line is, I still don't like it. But I drink at least six glasses a day, because I've become keenly aware of its benefits.

Bob and I would take long runs while training for the marathon. We would always pack plenty of water. I'd drink some every mile or so—thirsty or not. It certainly helped the workout. I could immediately feel the difference in my performance if my body had enough water. In addition, when I first started this program and I needed to lose a lot of weight, I noticed I was more successful dropping pounds if I followed the six-glass-minimum rule.

Following this step allowed me to drop weight more readily. I picture it this way: The water is flushing fat cells out of my body along with toxins and waste. I know that's not exactly the scientific explanation, but it works for me.

I also noticed a difference in my complexion. I have oily skin. I had been prone to breakouts, even at age 40! These occur less often the more water I drink. I have a glass before I work out, two right after. I carry a sixteen-ounce bottle of water on the set during tapings of the show. During every commercial break, I take a few sips. By the end of the show, I've had two more glasses. I'll have a glass with either lunch or dinner, and I've satisfied this step. Now on some days, I'll even have some bonus glasses.

When I first started this regimen, I made so many trips to the bathroom, I thought something was wrong with my kidneys. My body was just not accustomed to receiving that much water. For a long time my routine

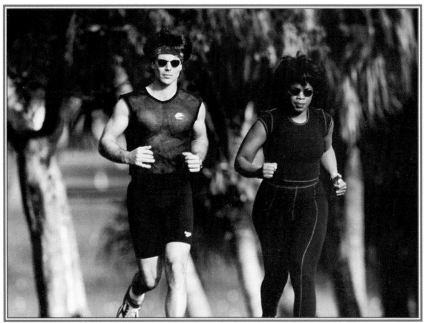

© TIM DE FRISCO 1996

was to drink and pee. So I made sure that I was never too far from a bathroom. Although once I was on a long run, with Bob, on a country road in Indiana. I had to stop four times and there was no place but cornfields and bushes. Bob would stand guard, while I made the best of it, four times. Each time I thought, if someone's hiding in the bushes and gets a picture of this, they'll never have to work again.

My body has adjusted better now, although I still don't drink water past six o'clock P.M., otherwise I'm making potty trips all night. And although I'll try water every imaginable way, I still don't like it. So I just count 'em down!

—Oprah

SOME of you will insist that you can't drink six to eight glasses of water every day. I've had people tell me that water has a bland taste, and others say that water has no taste. They say it's boring and that water is the last thing they crave. On the other hand, some of you will wonder why I even made this a step, since you naturally drink that much water each day.

When you see how water can help you lose weight, I think you will want to drink even more of it. Like all the steps, you will eventually come to perform this one out of habit. The more water you drink, the more your body will crave it. You may even get to the point where water is the first thing you want to drink in the morning. You might find that only water can quench your thirst.

Water is essential to life. Without it, we would survive maybe two to three days. That makes it our most important nutrient. Water surrounds and is a part of each and every cell in your body, and it's needed or involved in virtually all body functions. About 60 percent of your body weight is water.

We lose a lot of water each day through basic body functions. By exercising, you lose even more water depending on the type, length, and intensity of exercise and the climate you work out in. Your body must continually regulate the amount of water that it holds. You become dehydrated when your body's water supply cannot meet its demands. This can cause a variety of complications, including heat exhaustion and heat stroke. Although less life threatening, dehydration also affects the body's ability to digest food and metabolize fat. Needless to say, having enough water is essential for your body to function at its optimum.

As far as weight loss and weight maintenance are concerned, drinking enough water is extremely important. There are at least six basic reasons why replacing water on a daily basis is important for controlling your weight.

1. *Digestion and metabolism*—These are two functions we are particularly concerned with when it comes to controlling our weight. If you aren't getting enough water, you risk impairing these two functions to a certain degree. Enough water ensures that both digestion and metabolism are working at their full capacity.

2. *Water's filling effect*—By drinking six to eight glasses of water, you can help curb your appetite. Water can fill you up so that you don't overeat.

3. *The thirst-hunger response*—When you are dehydrated, your body may signal you to eat when what it really requires is water. It does the same thing for a variety of nutritional needs. For example, your body may need sodium, so it signals you to eat foods containing salt. But all you really need is the salt without all the additional calories in food. I call this phenomenon artificial hunger. By meeting all of your nutritional needs, including your need for water, you can control artificial hunger.

4. *Better workouts*—You can exercise more effectively and at higher levels when you are getting enough water.

5. *Muscle requires more water*—Muscle is comprised of about 70 percent water, whereas fat is made up of less than 25 percent water. One of the many benefits of exercise is that you maintain and even add muscle weight, which in turn burns fat. As you gain muscle, you require more water and need to replace more of it daily. So water becomes more important the more active you are. Think of it as a cycle: The more muscle you maintain, the more water is held by the body and the more calories are burned by that additional muscle. So the more muscle you have, the more water you must have available.

6. *Glycogen storage*—Glycogen is a form of carbohydrate stored in your muscles. It can be used as energy when you exercise. The more fit you become, the more glycogen is stored in your muscles. Every

gram of glycogen holds about 2.5 to 3 grams of water. So, the more fit you are, the more water your body will hold, and the more water you need each day. Being more fit also allows you to burn calories at a higher rate.

In addition to those six reasons, as you begin to lose fat, your body increases its percentage of water. So the amount of water you need to drink each day increases. This is especially so the more active you become. Your body is signaled to hold more water. It will usually let you know it needs more water by making you thirsty, but not always.

Just about all of the body's systems are regulated with amazing accuracy. One exception is our thirst mechanism. It is simply not perfect. By the time we experience thirst, our bodies are already in a slight state of dehydration. In addition, when our thirst is satisfied we may still be somewhat dehydrated. It is important to drink water throughout the day. It is also important to drink moderate-sized portions (one or two eight-ounce glasses) of water spread over the course of the day, rather than drink your six to eight glasses all at once. When we drink large quantities of water at one time, we stimulate the body to rid itself of water.

Until recently I considered carbonated (sparkling) water an acceptable source, but because of its diuretic effect, it should not be used to fulfill this step.

Although we get water from three primary sources, Step Eight requires you to drink six to eight glasses of water a day. This ensures that you are getting enough water. Don't worry about getting too much water, as your body will get rid of the excess. The sources are:

1. *Drinking liquids*—We receive water obviously by drinking it. We also receive water from juices, milk, soda, and essentially from all liquids that we drink. But these other liquids are not counted toward satisfying this step.

2. *The foods we eat*—Almost all foods contain water. The largest amount of water in foods is found in fruits and vegetables.

3. *Metabolic water*—When we break down an energy source, such as food or glycogen, we produce carbon dioxide and water. This water can, in turn, be used by your body.

I hope I have convinced you of the importance of drinking water, not just for your body's functions but for the weight-loss process as well. If you are still thinking it will be difficult to drink that much water and you are wondering how much you will be running to the bathroom, realize that over time your body will adjust. This step becomes easier the more active you are. And you will become more active!

Here's a perfect water day:

Start your day with a glass of water before your workout. You should be thirsty after your workout, so have two more glasses. You are already halfway toward your daily goal and it's still morning! Have another glass before or during lunch. Have another glass between lunch and dinner. Then finish off your day with a glass at dinner. This makes a total of six glasses. As you become more active, you might consider moving up to seven or eight glasses by adding more water either before or after your workout.

Tips

► EVEN THOUGH WATER IS FOUND IN OTHER BEVERAGES, YOU NEED TO CONSUME SIX TO EIGHT GLASSES OF FRESH WATER EACH DAY.

► TRY TO LIMIT THE AMOUNT OF CAFFEINE YOU CONSUME, SINCE CAFFEINE IS A STRONG DIURETIC AND STIMULATES YOUR BODY TO RELEASE WATER. IF YOU DRINK TEA OR ICED TEA, TRY HERBAL TEA. THIS WILL NOT COUNT TOWARD YOUR SIX TO EIGHT GLASSES, BUT IT DOES NOT CONTAIN CAFFEINE, AND IT'S HEALTHIER FOR YOU.

► MAKE WATER AVAILABLE TO YOURSELF AT ALL TIMES. THIS MAY INVOLVE CARRYING A BOTTLE OF WATER WITH YOU.

► TRY DIFFERENT BRANDS OF UNCARBONATED BOTTLED WATER. PICK YOUR FAVORITE!

► PLAY AROUND WITH THE TIMES YOU DRINK AS WELL AS THE AMOUNTS TO FIND A SYSTEM THAT WORKS FOR YOU.

► TRY TO AVOID DRINKING WATER LATE IN THE EVENING SINCE THIS WILL ONLY CAUSE YOU TO WAKE UP DURING THE NIGHT!

► GET INTO THE HABIT OF DRINKING ONE GLASS OF WATER FIRST THING IN THE MORNING. DRINK ANOTHER TWO AFTER YOUR WORKOUT.

► BE SURE YOUR GLASS OF WATER IS AESTHETICALLY PLEASING. USE AN ATTRACTIVE GLASS AND ADD LEMON OR LIME. DRESS IT UP!

Step Nine

HAVE AT LEAST TWO SERVINGS OF FRUIT AND THREE

SERVINGS OF VEGETABLES EACH DAY

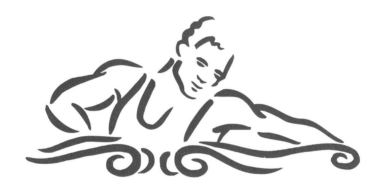

I've been consciously eating low-fat foods for about five years now. When I first started, I was bored, bored, bored by both fruits and vegetables. Because I'd done all the diets, fad and otherwise, I was familiar with the steamed broccoli, apple for a snack, celery and carrot sticks in the fridge routines. Boring!

Now I know there's a whole world of fruits and vegetables waiting to be discovered. One of my new favorite meals just happens to be a warm vegetable salad—which includes all my favorite vegetables—zucchini, eggplant, corn, tomatoes, peas—warmed and spread over lettuce. Who would have thought that would be one of my favorites five years ago? Not I!

As for fruits, all my life I ate what most people eat—apples, oranges, maybe grapes thrown in for some variety. I still eat these, but I've expanded my fruit awareness and developed some new favorites. Mango and papaya lead that list. Perfectly ripened honeydew can also make me want to sing a happy song.

I now like fruit for a pre-exercise snack. Often for dessert, I'll do a combination of fruits—strawberries, blueberries, and mango with a spoonful of frozen yogurt. So good it makes me want to tell somebody!

It's amazing how your tastes will change when you make it a habit to begin eating healthily. This step is a real good start.

—Oprah

I'M one to talk. I avoided fruits and vegetables most of my life, at least until I finished college. Then I discovered that I liked the taste of fruits. It wasn't for another eight years that I got onboard with vegetables. Once I did, I felt healthier, had more energy, became more fit, and, yes, lowered my percentage of body fat. Now, I love fruits and vegetables. You will too.

Fruits and vegetables are rich in nutrients. They contain water, vitamins, fiber, and minerals. And they are an essential part of good nutrition and sensible eating. You can accomplish so much just by eating two fruits and at least three vegetables each day.

First off, by fulfilling this step, you are all but assured to reach your recommended daily allowance (RDA) for many vitamins and minerals. In addition, the weight-loss value is high since there are relatively few calories in fruits and vegetables. They are also very satisfying and filling. So by filling up on them, you are less likely to eat unhealthy foods. And if I haven't sold you on fruits and vegetables yet, let me tell you that the health benefits go way beyond weight control. Recent studies support that eating at least five fruits and vegetables can reduce the risk of several forms of cancer. I think I've made my point: Eat at least two fruits and at least three vegetables each day!

Many people consider fruits and vegetables as one group, but there are differences between them. Let's first talk about fruits.

Fruits contain fructose. Fructose is a simple sugar, which is easily converted to body fat. So why would I be asking you to eat fruit? The answer is that fruits also contain many important nutrients as mentioned above. The benefits of eating fruit far outweigh any negatives. And you may recall from the food pyramid that they are an important component in a well-rounded nutrition plan.

Some fruits are better than others since they vary in their sugar, vitamin, mineral, water, and fiber content. The best fruits to eat include:

- Strawberries
- Apples (green apples contain the least sugar)
- Blueberries
- Grapefruit (including grapefruit juice)
- Pears

- Oranges
- Boysenberries
- Papaya
- Cranberries (including cranberry juice but not cranberry sauce)
- Blackberries
- Guava
- Cantaloupe

All fruits can and should be eaten from time to time, but the following is a list of fruits that are higher in sugar content and, therefore, calories and should be eaten less frequently.

- Coconut (also contains a fair amount of fat)
- Bananas (still a good snack and great with cereal)
- Grapes
- Dates
- Canned and processed fruit
- Dried fruit

Some basic tips about eating fruit

► FRUIT MAKES A GREAT SNACK.

► FRUIT IS A TERRIFIC "STARTER" SNACK PRIOR TO YOUR MORNING WORKOUT.

► RAW FRUIT IS BEST BUT IF FRUIT IS TO BE COOKED, BAKED OR STEAMED IS BETTER THAN BOILED. BOILING FRUIT LOWERS ITS NUTRITIONAL VALUE.

► FRUIT JUICE COUNTS AS A FRUIT. FOR ADDED FIBER, DRINK FRUIT JUICE WITH THE PULP.

Vegetables are a nutritional bonanza. Like fruits, they are rich in vitamins, minerals, water, and fiber. Vegetables have an additional benefit over fruits, however. They are a complex carbohydrate and thus cannot be converted to fat as easily as a simple sugar. Also, vegetables tend to be lower in total calories than fruits.

Vegetables are a critical part of a sound nutrition program. Of course when I speak of eating vegetables, I am referring to eating fresh vegetables that are either raw or steamed without oil or butter. Salads should be eaten without the use of high-fat salad dressings. Eating vegetables in this manner can help you tremendously in reaching your ideal weight. This will also lower your risk for various cancers and heart disease. I could go on and on about the benefits of eating vegetables. Instead I'll simply say: Eat at least three a day and consider eating four, five, or even six if you like!

The best vegetables to eat include:

- Alfalfa sprouts
- Artichokes
- Broccoli
- Brussels sprouts
- Cabbage
- Carrot
- Celery
- Collard greens
- Eggplant
- Green beans
- Kale
- Leeks
- Mushrooms
- Okra
- Lettuce
- Onions
- Scallions

- Spinach
- Summer squash
- Tomato
- Turnips
- Turnip greens
- Watercress
- Zucchini

The following vegetables should be limited or avoided:

- Avocado (high in fat)
- Canned, processed, or frozen vegetables

If you are not accustomed to eating fruits and vegetables in the recommended daily amounts, you may have trouble at first getting into the habit. As you begin adopting a healthy diet and an active lifestyle, your body will naturally crave fruits and vegetables. So, as always, just be patient!

Some basic tips about eating vegetables

➤ VEGETABLES CAN AND SHOULD BE COMBINED WITH FOODS SUCH AS BROWN RICE AND PASTA TO CREATE EXCITING MEALS.

➤ ONE OR TWO VEGETABLES SHOULD ALWAYS BE EATEN AT DINNER.

➤ RAW VEGETABLES ARE GREAT SNACKS. THEY ARE ACTUALLY THE BEST SNACK. FOR EXAMPLE, CARROT STICKS, CELERY STICKS, RAW BROCCOLI, OR RAW CAULIFLOWER.

➤ VEGETABLES ARE BEST RAW, STEAMED, OR GRILLED AS OPPOSED TO BOILED OR FRIED.

➤ VEGETABLES NEED LITTLE OR NO OIL IN THEIR PREPARATION. IF YOU ARE ACCUSTOMED TO USING OIL, GRADUALLY REDUCE THE AMOUNT YOU USE.

➤ TRY EATING MORE VEGETABLES AT TIMES YOU NORMALLY WOULDN'T. TRY THEM FOR BREAKFAST, LUNCH, AND SNACKS.

Step Ten

RENEW YOUR COMMITMENT TO HEALTHY
LIVING EACH DAY (DAILY RENEWAL)

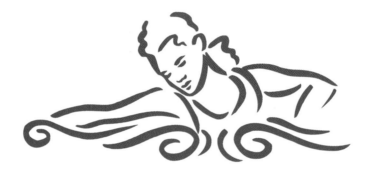

I remember a day, back in 1995, almost a year after I ran the Marine Corps Marathon. I was in the seventh lap, around a six-lap-per-mile indoor track. I had 23 laps to go to complete my five-mile run for the day. I wondered why the run that day was so difficult. It wasn't even 6 A.M. yet, but I felt like I'd been exercising all day. Was it that my breathing was off, or the fact that I had two oak stumps faking as legs that prevented me from moving faster than a 9.37-per-minute mile? "Every step is a struggle," I declared to Bob. "Why does it have to be so hard for me—it never gets any easier!" I added. I was ready to stop, put my fist through the wall, and have a good scream. "I can't believe it's this hard for everyone. Struggle, struggle, struggle. It never ends." By this time I was literally screaming.

"Why do you look at it as a struggle?" Bob answered calmly—running his usual three steps ahead. "Why don't you change the way you think about the whole process? Think of it as renewing yourself each day. This is what it feels like. And this is what it takes. It's going to be harder some days than others, but on any given day, your body gives you what it has. Just do the best you can. This is what you have to work with today. This is today's daily renewal."

At that moment, lights and bells went off for me. Ding! Ding! Ding! That was the jackpot, breakthrough, answer for me. He was right! I was doing the best I could, given what I had that day. I also realized that I had done the best I could over the past two and a half years and it had allowed me to accomplish what I never could before. I was happy with my efforts and myself. The effort that I put forth each day is what it takes for me to stay in shape and to feel good. The only question was, was I willing on a daily basis to do what it took? For the first time in my life, knowing all that it takes, I can honestly say—yes.

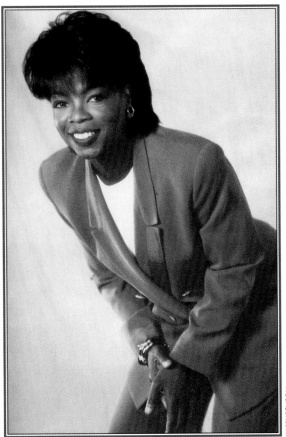

HARRY BENSON

People often ask me what keeps me motivated to work out and eat right each day. I often jokingly respond, "I don't want my fat butt back." Although that's partially true, the real answer is that I never want to be anesthetized by the extra weight again. For me, overeating, not working out, and the inevitable weight gain that followed was my way of repressing, stifling emotions, procrastinating pain and discomfort, and avoiding my true feelings.

The truth is that in spite of all my professional success, I now realize that I've spent a lifetime being afraid. Afraid of not being liked. Afraid of hurting people's feelings. Afraid of confrontation. Afraid of being used. Afraid of expressing love.

True love begins with yourself. You can give and give and give to other people. Care for them, nurture them, support them. But it's the support and care and love that you give yourself that gives you the real strength to care for and love others. This has been a long and difficult lesson for me to learn, but I'm finally getting it.

Each day I put forth the effort to take care of myself, work out, eat healthy food, deal with my feelings and not bury them in a giant bag of Dorito's, confront people when necessary, tell people the truth, and tell myself the truth. This has changed my life—I have been freed from my own personal prison.

I feel free. Free to live in the moment. Free to enjoy everyone I can. When pain, betrayal, judgment, or adversity come—I live that too. I can face it straight up and know that it, too, shall pass—every moment does. I'm no longer afraid. I am more connected to myself.

It's been a long time coming for me. This is not an easy journey to take. As a matter of fact, ridding yourself of the weight and all that the weight represents may be one of the most difficult things you can do. It can also be one of the most rewarding—it has been for me. No doubt some of you are where I was three years ago. You've tried everything, failed many times over, and you think nothing will work. You have to change your perception. It's not about weight, it's about caring for yourself on a daily basis. Renew! Renew! Renew!

The ten steps will move you toward making the connection.

—**Oprah**

EVEN if you faithfully follow the ten steps, you can't expect to have perfect days every day of the year. You will have perfect days, you will have good days, you will have mediocre days, and you will have downright awful days. Just as in life. But the beauty of daily renewal is that no matter how yesterday went, you have the opportunity to improve on it and better yourself today. Step ten is the most important step for helping you manage your weight for the rest of your life. I saved this step for last. But it will be the first step you perform each day.

Renewing yourself every day is more than a step. It is a philosophy—an outlook on life. It is reminding yourself each day that you are alive and that there is so much you want to accomplish in your life. It confirms what is truly important to you. Obviously this step reaches way beyond the goal of losing weight. But then, this book has always been about more than losing weight.

Daily renewal is a statement about how you wish your day and, ultimately, your life to unfold. It is your soul speaking to your heart, your heart translating to your mind, and your mind giving your body directions. It is ultimately an expression of self-love!

One of the goals in this step is to show you that you have control over the events in your life. But in order to gain control, you first need to know yourself, then you need to know what you want. You need to take responsibility for all things in your life, and finally you need to remind yourself each day of your goals and what you are going to do to work toward them. This is what daily renewal is all about. This step can lead you to self-acceptance and, finally, to self-love.

The key to this step is performing it each day. Daily renewal begins when you first wake up. You take a few moments to state what is important to you, what you wish to accomplish, and the steps you will take that day to work toward your goals. These can be long-term goals or immediate ones. They can be goals pertaining to your body and health, or simply anything you wish to accomplish. For example, you wake up in the morning and announce to yourself: "I want to care more about myself, and I am willing to do what it takes to achieve that. Today, that means I will follow all ten steps. That will be my gift to myself." Starting out, you may decide it's best to write down your renewal statement. Later you may say it out loud or just say it to yourself—whatever works for you.

You will keep this statement in mind throughout the day, calling upon it especially when events and circumstances seem to challenge your true desires. Remember the commitment you made to yourself just that morning. It will give you strength.

Then, each evening, take the time to review how your day went. You can write down what happened in a journal. How could you have improved on this day? What went wrong, what went right, how will it be different tomorrow. Compliment yourself for great days. Vow to improve on days that weren't so great. Then, put that day to rest and set yourself up to renew again tomorrow.

It sounds so simple on paper. But there will be days that test your patience and will. On days you are able to meet the challenge, it is cause to praise yourself. On days you don't, give yourself the opportunity to improve.

To assist you in renewing yourself each day, I've already mentioned that a journal is useful. Before I met Oprah, I often encouraged my clients to use a log or journal. Even though it was basic—they stated their weight-loss goals and kept track of what they ate and when they exercised—they still found it quite useful. It also helped me evaluate how they were doing. Meeting Oprah, I was glad to hear that she had kept a journal for most of her adult life. From time to time, during workouts, she would recall stories from her journal, and I was always amazed by how much she detailed events and her feelings about them. Those details helped Oprah figure out when and why she ate.

Since working with her, I now think one of the most important aspects of a journal is accurately writing about your feelings. You can learn so much about yourself at the time you write, as well as later, when you look back to see how much you've changed. I now encourage clients to write with abandon about their feelings regarding themselves, food, exercise, motivation, and life in general. I also ask them to include their statement of daily renewal. This technique has been invaluable, and I highly recommend it to you.

A journal can also help you organize your performance of the other nine steps you will do each day. It's a good idea to maintain your journal for at least three months. After that time, all ten steps will have become part of your lifestyle and you will carry them out without much thought. Then, it's up to you whether you want to continue keeping a journal. Remember, your journal can be as individual as you are. To help you organize your journal, here's a list of things you can include:

- Your renewal statement for the day (be sure to state your goals and what you will do to work toward them)
- Your weekly weight, if you wish
- Your performance on each of the ten steps
    Your exercise routine, how long it was, and at what level
    Number of fat grams eaten
    Number of meals and snacks
    Number of alcoholic beverages consumed
    Time of your last meal and time you went to sleep
    How many glasses of water you drank
    Number of fruits and vegetables eaten
- Why and when you ate due to stress or emotions
- Your general feelings about food, exercise, life
- Any really good events or feelings you had during the day
- Your overall performance rating on how the day went
- Reflect on how your day went and how it can be improved tomorrow

Following is a sample journal entry:

Nov. 4 1995 5:30 Am

I'm still tired from yesterday's 6 mile run. My legs feel like two lead pipes It's going to be tough trying to maintain the 9:20 pace I've held all week. I'll do my best.

8:17pm I maintained well on the food side. I had 3 low fat cookies instead of 2, but I'm not gonna beat myself up about it. I drank so much water 8 full glasses — by the second show I had to stop tape twice for p break.

From somewhere I gathered strength today. Pulled it up from my thighs! I'm still amazed that I can stand the morning barely able to get out of bed — run 5 miles and actually feel better. Stopped eating at 7:00 pm. Gonna try and be 1 second faster tomorrow!

You can use a blank book or notebook, or you can purchase the Journal of Daily Renewal that Oprah and I have prepared in conjunction with this book. Either way, be sure to add any additional information you feel is helpful to you. You can keep your journal by your bed and log your entries at night, or carry it with you throughout the day and log events as they happen. It's up to you.

What I've just shared with you are the mechanics of daily renewal. But to really understand and benefit from daily renewal, you need to experience so much more. There are two concepts I want to introduce to you. They go hand-in-hand with daily renewal. They are:

1. Living in the moment

2. Finding joy in your life

I believe that without incorporating these two concepts into your day and your life, you will have a difficult time maintaining any results you achieve. More important, I can't imagine a fulfilling life without the feeling of living in the moment and experiencing true joy. Some of you may be familiar with these concepts. Some of you may think I'm speaking a foreign language.

When I first began working with people who wanted to lose weight or needed to improve their health for medical reasons, I never mentioned these concepts. I did, however, notice that all the people I worked with were preoccupied with either the past or the future. They never seemed to experience the present. Looking back, I realize that most of these people were never joyful. The two concepts are related. It is much easier to experience true joy when you learn to live "in the moment."

I also remember a time in my life when many wonderful things would happen, but I never took the time to appreciate them. Instead, I was always so focused on the future. I thought by doing that, more of these great things would happen. Now I realize, what's the point of good things in your life if they are never recognized or appreciated as they happen?

I'll never forget a moment about ten years ago. I was by myself, skiing in one of my favorite places on earth, Telluride, Colorado. Telluride has some of the most beautiful scenery in the world. Here I was, on a particular peak overlooking a valley. Past the valley, I could see the mountains of Utah. It was such an incredibly clear and beautiful day. The snow was a deep, fluffy powder. The sun was out. The air was crisp and fresh. And as I stood there, overlooking this incredible view, in one of my favorite places, doing one of my favorite things, I had the sudden realization: "I'm not happy."

For a moment I just stood there, staring out at that mountain range, trying to understand how it was that I was not happy. I couldn't figure out why. How could it be? I replayed that entire day, in particular the time I spent skiing. Then, it dawned on me. For that entire, beautiful day, I was mentally somewhere else. I was thinking about my career plans, buying a house, what day I was going home, whether my car would start since I had been gone for two weeks. I was preoccupied with everything that I was *going* to do, and not anything that I was *doing.*

I asked myself if I had appreciated one single moment of that day as it happened. Then I tried to remember the last time I appreciated any moment. I had to admit, it had been quite a while. This startled me enough to pop my skis off and sit down in the snow. I continued to stare at the mountains of Utah. It took me a while, but for the first time that day, I got into the current moment. I began to enjoy everything around me. It was peaceful. It was glorious. I'm not sure how long I sat in the snow, but time did not matter. It was a joyful moment.

Only after I experienced living in the moment was I able to experience true joy. How could I have been so preoccupied before? I wondered. I began questioning why most people focus on either the past or the future, when their entire life is lived in the present. I had to ask myself why I was always thinking of the future. The answer in all instances was that there was discontent with something about the present. That discontent was what made me obsess about improving my future. So in a sense, I was sacrificing my present for my future, not realizing that the future never really arrives. It's always the future! I decided from that day on that I was going to experience as many current moments as I could. Soon after that, I began experiencing the present moment on a regular basis, and true joy often followed. This has changed my life.

I began using this knowledge in my work, with great results. I found that almost everyone I worked with was not living in the moment, mainly due to the fact that they did not like something about the present, often something about themselves. When these same people learned to accept themselves and appreciate things about themselves right then and there, they were more easily able to live in the present. And they experienced "true joy" breakthroughs more frequently.

These are difficult concepts for people who struggle with weight, since they are often very unhappy with themselves. They usually believe they can only be happy and joyful when the weight is removed. This is almost never the case. If and when these same individuals reach their goal weight, they realize that they are still unhappy with themselves. And they almost always return to their old habits of eating poorly and not exercising to mask the pain.

I can't stress enough the importance of living in the moment, of experiencing each moment, both the good and bad moments that make up your life. This will open you up to feelings of true joy, and that's what life is all about. After all, true joy is an expression of love.

Will being in the moment open you up to sorrow and sadness? Yes, it will. As I'm sure you know, these are also part of life. Just remember that feeling sorrow and sadness will allow you to feel true joy to greater depths. Temporary setbacks are opportunities in disguise—opportunities to improve.

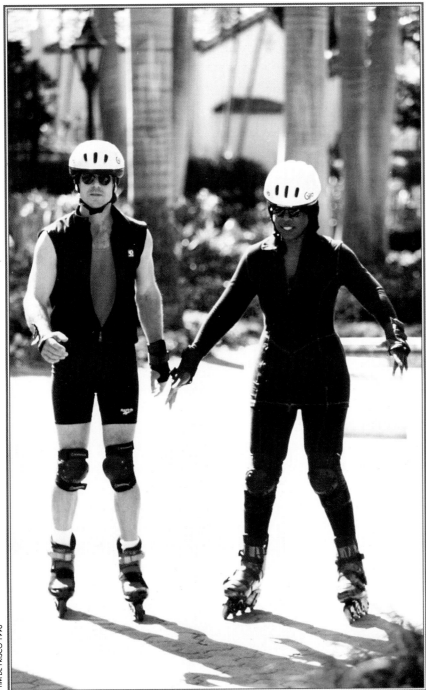

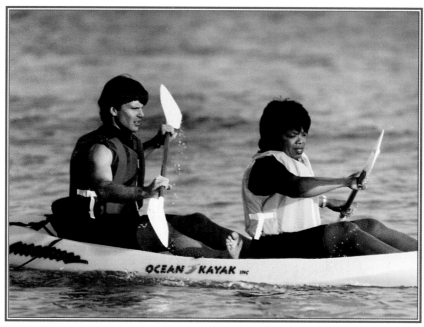

© TIM DE FRISCO 1996

So how do you begin to live in the moment and find true joy? This is really a spiritual question, and different people have taken various paths to experiencing and expressing love. You should select a path according to your own values and beliefs. But it can begin with just being conscious of the concept of living in the moment. Make an effort to experience real moments in each day. As you begin the process of self-acceptance, you should find that you are living in the moment more frequently. And you should certainly be able to recognize any feelings of true joy. By caring for yourself enough to read this book and adopt its principles, you have already begun the process.

Even exercising regularly will improve your ability to live in the moment. It is one the best teachers of this concept that I know. Let me explain. The task of exercising, especially at level seven or eight, forces you to be in the moment. As you will see, you can't help but

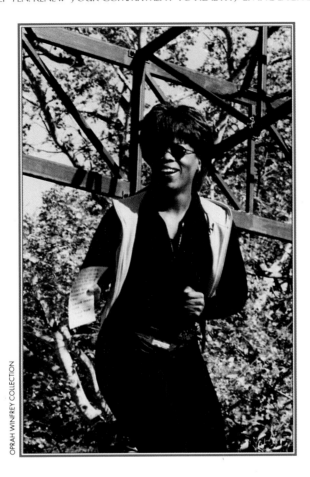

experience how you are feeling. You become very aware of your breathing, of every muscle that is working, how fatigued you are. You have little choice but to be in the moment. Just try thinking about the past or the future while you exercise! What I'm saying is, daily exercise forces you to focus on what you are experiencing. So you are living in the moment, at least for the duration of your workout session.

Exercise acts as a mini-course in living in the moment, a course you attend daily or almost daily. Once you begin experiencing living in the moment at least once a day, you are more likely to experience it at other times throughout the day. Eventually, you will find that you are living in the moment quite frequently. You may find that you want to try different things, things you never thought you would try.

Most recently this happened with some of the participants of the Get Movin' with Oprah Spring Training campaign. In the spring of 1995, Oprah did a series of shows and walks throughout the country to get people focused on fitness and eating right. Months after the campaign ended, she started getting phone calls and letters from some participants. Many of them mentioned how they were trying something new in their lives. They were taking up lessons for tennis, golf, and dance. They told me stories about going to various social functions, taking adventure trips, riding in hot air balloons, even hiking in the Himalayas. The descriptions of these events were almost always followed by the words: "I never would have done this before." I'm always thrilled to hear these stories, because I know there has been a real change in people's lives.

The same thing happened to Oprah. She now does all sorts of things she never dreamed she would do: running races, swimming, kayaking, jet-skiing, hiking the Grand Canyon, rollerblading, even riding an elephant to open the last show for the Get Movin' campaign. It's a very different life for her than it was three years ago. Your life will change as well.

You will also start feeling better about yourself, and that alone will help move you toward self-acceptance. Accepting yourself and living in the moment will increase your opportunities for experiencing true joy. When you have feelings of true joy on a regular basis, you are moving toward self-love. And that is a beautiful experience.

When I first met Oprah, I never saw her experience joy. I began watching her show and would catch glimpses of her expressing joy on the air. But I never saw it in real life. One day we were taking a long walk along Indiana's backroads when I thought to ask her about it. I had been working with her for only three or four months, so I wasn't sure how she would react to such a personal question. "How often do you feel joy in your life?" I asked. She appeared caught off guard. "What do you mean?" she stalled. I repeated my question. "How often do you experience real joy?" Now, she stopped in her tracks and said nothing. I then asked her when was the last time she'd experienced a joyful moment. "Ah. I'm trying to remember," she said. "Real joy. I think it was 1985, when I was doing *The Color Purple*. I loved every single moment of it." I dropped the subject, but her response made me sad. I could tell it made her sad too. Here it was 1993. She hadn't experienced real joy in almost eight years.

I thought of her typical day: taping two shows, reviewing those shows, making hundreds of decisions each day regarding the future of her company and her potential upcoming projects, sorting through the thousands of requests she gets each week. Her day was filled with lists of things to do, and she was always focused on what she had to do next. Her show was the exception. During that hour, she was occasionally able to live in the moment. But on top of everything, she was not happy about herself, mostly because her past was still a painful part of her present. With all the time she spent dealing with her past and focusing on her future, I could see she had little time to be in the present. No wonder she had so little joy in her life.

As time went on and Oprah was more successful with her weight-loss program, I began to see her express little bouts of happiness. I remember the first summer after I started working with her, we were out at her farm and she had a couple of girlfriends visiting. They were the perfect picture of Southern ladies, with their sundresses and wide-brimmed hats on, sitting on Oprah's porch, singing along to Bonnie Raitt songs. When I walked up to the porch to let Oprah know I was ready for our second workout of that day, she gave me an almost defiant look. "Bob, I've had the best day, and I'm not working out again today." She looked so genuinely happy that all I could say was, "Have fun." Two weeks later, Oprah was back at the farm with those same friends, and they were all wearing hats again. "Uh, oh," I joked.

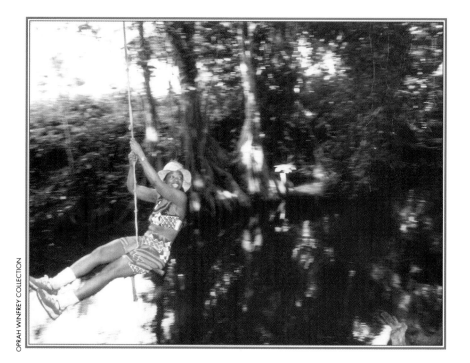

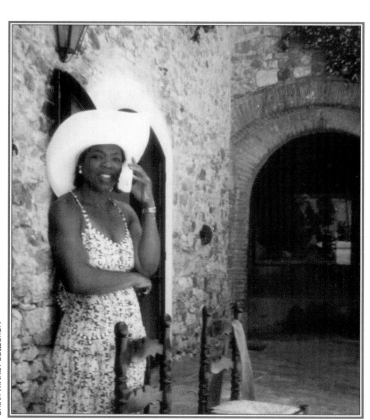

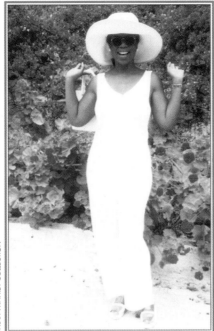

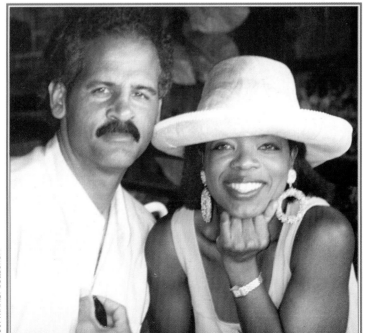

"Every time I see those hats, I know it means trouble." We all laughed. This time, though, Oprah was ready to work out.

She wore a hat many days that summer.

These joyful moments became more frequent and more intense. But her strongest joyful moment I ever witnessed came in October 1994. We had been running for over four hours in pouring rain during the Marine Corps Marathon in Washington, D.C. Oprah had run a perfect race. I looked up and saw the 25-mile marker. It was clear she would finish. I turned around, and I saw Oprah with tears in her eyes.

I immediately thought of the time when I first met her. She was 237 pounds and couldn't look me in the eye. I remembered all the obstacles she had overcome—her difficult childhood, her food addiction, her busy, stressful life—to be there that day. I recalled all of the hard work, self-discipline, desire, and commitment she showed over the last two years that prepared her for this race. I replayed so many memories of her journey. I thought of all the miles run on dusty Indiana backroads. I thought of her hiking the trails of Telluride. I thought of all the 5 A.M. workouts, the Grand Canyon, the hills of Umbria, and fried calamari. I thought about her wearing a hat and singing to Bonnie Raitt songs. I thought of her reaching her goal weight and wearing a size-eight dress. I thought of all the long runs when she was exhausted but kept going anyway.

And when I looked into her eyes brimming with tears, I knew she was replaying those memories too. I had never seen her so joyful. It was an unforgettable moment.

What Oprah experienced was the culminating moment in a journey that began with her knowing herself, taking responsibility for who and what she was, knowing what she wanted, working hard for it, accepting herself, living in the moment, and feeling joy. At that moment, she was expressing love.

And, you know, that's exactly why we're here.